"The information in *Eating Right for a Bad Gut* has had a major impact on my approach to the dietary management of IBD, both as a doctor and a patient."
　　　　　　　—From the Foreword by R. Balfour Sartor, M.D.

"Dr. Scala has introduced a whole new era in the alleviation of symptoms of IBD. . . . Well-researched, easy to read . . . a *must* for anyone involved with this problem."
　　　　　　　—Dr. Bruce B. Miller, president, Diet Analysis Center

"FRANK AND CONCISE . . . Scala provides straightforward recommendations for healthy eating that's easy on the gut. . . . He knows his subject well and always comes across as hopeful and helpful—without preaching."　　　　　*—Publishers Weekly*

"OFFERS WAYS TO GET LASTING RELIEF through proper diet, exercise and stress management." *—Rocky Mountain News*

DR. JAMES SCALA has been involved witʰ and health research for over twenty year ed with both Shaklee Corporation aⁿ s an elected member of the A American Institute of Nu Nutrition, and the British s taught nutrition and/or biochemist ⁿ Medical School, the University of Oklahoma al School, the Ohio College of Medicine, and the University of California at Berkeley. His previous books include *The Arthritis Relief Diet* and *The High Blood Pressure Relief Diet* (available in NAL Books and Plume editions). He lives in Lafayette, California.

Other Books by James Scala

Making the Vitamin Connection
The Arthritis Relief Diet
The High Blood Pressure Relief Diet

EATING RIGHT FOR A BAD GUT

The Complete Nutritional Guide to ILEITIS, COLITIS, CROHN'S DISEASE AND INFLAMMATORY BOWEL DISEASE

DR. JAMES SCALA

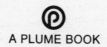

A PLUME BOOK

NOTE TO THE READER
The ideas, procedures, and suggestions contained in this book are not intended as a substitute for consulting with your physician. All matters regarding your health require medical supervision.

PLUME
Published by the Penguin Group
Penguin Books USA Inc., 375 Hudson Street, New York, New York 10014, U.S.A.
Penguin Books Ltd, 27 Wrights Lane, London W8 5TZ, England
Penguin Books Australia Ltd, Ringwood, Victoria, Australia
Penguin Books Canada Ltd, 10 Alcorn Avenue, Toronto, Ontario, Canada M4V 3B2
Penguin Books (N.Z.) Ltd, 182-190 Wairau Road, Auckland 10, New Zealand

Penguin Books Ltd, Registered Offices: Harmondsworth, Middlesex, England

Published by Plume, an imprint of New American Library, a division of Penguin Books USA Inc.
Previously published in an NAL Books edition.

First Plume Printing, January, 1992
10 9 8 7 6 5 4 3 2 1

 REGISTERED TRADEMARK—MARCA REGISTRADA

LIBRARY OF CONGRESS CATALOGING-IN-PUBLICATION DATA
Scala, James, 1934-
    Eating right for a bad gut : the complete nutritional guide to
ileitis, colitis, Crohn's disease, and inflammatory bowel disease /
James Scala.
        p.   cm.
    Includes bibliographical references and index.
    ISBN 0-452-26766-8
    1. Inflammatory bowel diseases—Popular works.   2. Inflammatory
bowel diseases—Diet therapy.   3. Inflammatory bowel diseases—
Nutritional aspects.   I. Title.
[RC862.I53S23   1992]
616.3'440654—dc20   91-34998
                                                         CIP

Printed in the United States of America
Original hardcover design by Leonard Telesca

To people with inflammatory bowel disease:

Through your thoughts, questions, ideas, and encouragement, you helped me write this book; it's your book.

—James Scala

Contents

PART TWO

PART THREE

APPENDIX

Acknowledgments

Many people made this book possible. They all were willing to help whenever asked.

Special thanks goes to my wife, Nancy, for the many hours she put in typing, talking to people, seeking information, and spending many a tea break discussing the illness.

My daughters, Kim and Nancy, for their general help in typing, photocopying, and running to the library when asked.

Al Zuckerman for his positive attitude in selling the concept.

Alexia Dorszynski for her support, patience, and for always being there when I needed her.

Judy Kuo, my favorite teenage typist, for her ability to translate my longhand into a nicely typed format. Her conscientiousness is eclipsed only by her pleasant smile.

I am indebted to the many people who filled out questionnaires, wrote letters regarding their disease, and talked openly about living with Inflammatory Bowel Disease. They provided me with valuable information that will be a real service to other individuals with the disease. I'm most grateful for their willingness to be so frank, sincere, and genuinely interested. My heartfelt thanks!

R. Balfour Sartor, M.D., for graciously reading the manuscript and generously giving me the benefit of his knowledge.

Last, but certainly not least, my family for their encouragement and understanding of the long hours and weekends spent writing and editing.

Foreword

By conservative estimates, between 500,000 and 800,000 adults and children in the United States suffer from ulcerative colitis or Crohn's disease (ileitis). The cause of these related disorders, collectively referred to as inflammatory bowel disease (IBD), is unknown, and medical therapy suppresses, but does not cure, the inflammation. Even surgery, which can cure ulcerative colitis at the expense of removing the entire colon (large intestine), is only of temporary help to patients with Crohn's disease, who have a very high postoperative recurrence rate. In spite of these sobering characteristics, the majority of patients with IBD adapt to their symptoms and maintain productive lives.

Dietary management can dramatically improve the cardinal symptoms of diarrhea, abdominal pain, and weight loss. Most patients and their families constantly experiment with their diet and gradually, by trial and error, discover which foods can be tolerated and which produce worsened symptoms, frequently misinterpreted as a "flare-up" of their disease. All too frequently, IBD patients will mistakenly eliminate many important foods from their diet because that food was associated with abdominal pain or diarrhea on one occasion, thereby ending up on a diet deficient in many essential nutrients. In many cases, the entire family also adopts the restrictive diet of the patient for convenience.

This book is designed to take the guesswork out of nutrition by presenting general principles for a healthy diet for all family members while providing easily managed guidelines to the creation of an individualized dietary program aimed at diminishing symptoms, preventing complications, and optimizing function for the patient with ulcerative colitis or Crohn's disease.

Because IBD has no medical cure, dietary management assumes an essential role in the treatment plan. Eighty-five percent of Crohn's disease patients experience weight loss, and many children with IBD fail to grow because of decreased food consumption brought on by lack of appetite and increased abdominal pain and diarrhea after eating. Medications commonly used to treat IBD cause excessive losses of calcium and potassium, which, when combined with decreased absorption and increased loss of protein, vitamins, and minerals by the inflamed intestine, lead to severe malnutrition and vitamin deficiency states that complicate surgery and diminish a patient's energy level. The best therapy is prevention of such nutritional complications and enhancement of function by consuming a prudent balanced diet with vitamin and mineral supplementation, while avoiding foods that reproducibly produce increased symptoms. Most experienced physicians believe that the well-nourished patient with IBD responds more completely to medications and avoids many complications that may require surgery.

Dr. James Scala's *Eating Right for a Bad Gut* presents an overall health plan of diet, exercise, and stress management that is complementary to medical therapy and assists patients with IBD and their families to take an active role in the management of these chronic disorders. Drawing upon his extensive knowledge of nutrition and the effects of intestinal inflammation and medications on nutrient absorption, as well as a survey of over a hundred patients with Crohn's disease and ulcerative colitis, Dr. Scala provides an entertaining yet complete review of the fundamentals of nutrition and presents a dietary management plan tailored to the specific needs of IBD patients. His conversational writing style and references to historical notes, folk remedies, and native custom provide enjoyable yet very educational reading. The information and insight I gathered from this book have had a major impact on my approach to the dietary management of IBD, both as a gastroenterologist primarily treating patients with IBD and as a patient myself, coping with Crohn's disease for twenty years.

—R. Balfour Sartor, M.D.
Associate Professor of Medicine
Department of Digestive Diseases and Nutrition
School of Medicine
University of North Carolina at Chapel Hill

Preface

"Let Food Be Thy Medicine"
—HIPPOCRATES, ca. 450 B.C.

Chronic Illness

A chronic illness is an illness that doesn't leave; it's always there, even if it's not active (in remission). Inflammatory diseases, such as arthritis, psoriasis, and inflammatory bowel syndrome, are good examples of such illnesses. Once you have one of these diseases, it becomes part of your life. For instance, a person with rheumatoid arthritis may feel fine most of the time, yet a weather change can cause knees or other joints to start aching; or a serious, stressful event can cause joints to swell so badly that walking becomes difficult. Or the arthritis might require medication every day and never go into remission.

IBD—A Chronic Illness

Once it's established that you have IBD—Inflammatory Bowel Disease—you are a member of a small group who have

1

a chronic inflammatory illness. IBD is an inflammatory disease of the intestinal tract. When it flares up, the intestine becomes swollen; in some cases, sores develop, and sometimes they bleed. However, IBD can go into remission as a result of good medical care and a judicious diet. By practicing proper dietary care and avoiding stress during remission, life can be completely normal with only minor diarrhea to remind you that the disease is still there. Nevertheless, you can't be too complacent, because IBD can flare up so badly that the only safe treatment is hospitalization; sometimes aggressive surgery is necessary to remove part of the intestinal tract. And even after surgery, the illness is not gone; it's still a part of you. You'll have to watch your diet and take care to avoid things that can cause the problem to flare up.

Medication and Diet

Chronic illness often requires daily medication and a healthful diet. Too often people with a chronic illness take medication and assume that they don't need to watch their diet. Nothing could be more incorrect; diet can *always* be used to optimize life. Chronic illness makes diet more important. Proper diet can help reduce the need for medication and can help make life more satisfying.

What Is IBD?

Inflammatory bowel disease, or IBD, is the overall name given to diseases that attack the bowel wall, causing inflammation. Your doctor may call the disease by a number of terms, including colitis, proctitis, enteritis, and ileitis; however, you'll probably be told you either have ulcerative colitis, colitis, or Crohn's disease. In this book I will simply refer to all of them as IBD.

Ulcerative colitis is an IBD that causes ulcers, open sores, and inflammation of the large intestine. It almost always causes bloody, watery stools and involves the rectum. Ulcerative colitis can involve most of the large intestine beginning at the anus. When the entire organ is involved, there are seldom any areas that aren't inflamed and ulcerated. The disease doesn't cause other symptoms in other parts of the body. Plain *colitis* doesn't involve ulcerations and seems to be confined more to the upper part of the large intestine. When it's found adjacent to the ileum, it's sometimes called Crohn's colitis. If you want more detail, I suggest you read one of the publications listed in the Suggested Reading section at the end of the book.

Crohn's disease is characterized by inflammation that spreads deep into the bowel wall and is usually confined to one or more segments of the small intestine, especially the lower portion, or ileum. In about 50 percent of cases, it includes both the ileum and the first part of the large intestine, the colon. About 20 percent of cases involve only the colon.

Symptoms of IBD

Whether it involves the large or small intestine, IBD produces diarrhea and serious abdominal pain. Both Crohn's and colitis cause rectal bleeding. Ulcerative colitis is the only one that usually causes serious bleeding, however. If the bleeding persists, the loss of blood can lead to anemia—a shortage of red blood cells. In IBD, red blood cells can be lost in the blood faster than your body can make them.

Intestinal inflammation can result in poor absorption of nutrients; the diarrhea causes an actual loss of nutrients. Together, these symptoms can cause weight loss and poor nutrition. If inflammation persists, it can require medical treatment, because the person who has it is actually suffering from poor nutrition.

Symptoms of IBD are not always confined to the intestine and can appear in other places: sores in the mouth, similar to small canker sores; inflammation of the eyes; arthritis inflammation, usually in one joint, such as a knee or wrist; ulcerlike sores and red nodules on the skin, especially the abdomen and legs. The red nodules aren't powerful, but the ulcers can become infected. Sometimes these added symptoms precede the intestinal involvement. In fact, these other symptoms are often a warning that IBD is about to flare up.

IBD in Children

About 20 percent of the adults with IBD exhibit symptoms before age 15. The disease is rarely diagnosed before age 10, as in 25 percent of all cases, unless, another family member has the disease. When another family member has IBD, early diagnosis is more likely. IBD can also be diagnosed in children under age 4, however; one major clue is that the child begins to fall behind peers in development. IBD is not easy to diagnose in children, because like many illnesses, it starts slowly and builds. Consequently, it's not uncommon for the pediatrician to consider other illnesses, such as an intestinal flu, or even anorexia.

Because of the symptoms, a doctor could justifiably suspect that emotional problems are the cause of cramps or anorexia. The child associates food with discomfort; hence, the child logically learns not to eat. (If you ate and got sick, you'd cut back on eating, too.) By not eating properly, the child reduces calories and nutrient-intake and stunts its growth. This developmental lag often causes confusion of the true illness, IBD, with other illnesses.

Most physicians agree that children with IBD must eat— their bodies need calories for growth. They also need to eat foods that don't cause discomfort. Fortunately, they can use supplements and supplemental foods to get their nutrition (see Chapters Seven and Eight).

Children with IBD can fail to thrive from lack of nourishment. They experience poor growth and development. This slow growth is a problem, because after puberty is complete, they can't make up for the shortfall. But that's not all. If absorption of a nutrient, such as zinc, is reduced, the physical development of some organs will be delayed and might even be incomplete for life. Poor nutrition in children is tragic and is a major reason why physicians keep a close watch on children with IBD. Nothing can be left to chance.

Flare-ups

Since IBD is a chronic disease, once you've got it, you've always got it, even if a period of remission is so complete there are no symptoms. IBD can go into remission for years, and during these periods of remission, life seems to be normal except for some diarrhea and occasional discomfort. Persons who have IBD, however, always seem to have watery stools, although dietary fiber and some medications can help to relieve that problem. And diarrhea is a minor discomfort compared to other aspects of the disease.

The return of IBD with all its symptoms is called a flare-up. Flare-ups characterize other inflammatory diseases, such as arthritis, psoriasis, asthma, and others; we'll discuss the comparison to these illnesses shortly. At this point, let me just say that a flare-up represents a serious return of symptoms. The term *flare-up* covers a wide range of symptoms, from a return of abdominal cramps and diarrhea to the need for hospitalization. The flare-up can be so serious and long lasting that total parenteral nutrition—TPN—is required, meaning that the patient is fed entirely through a major vein and the digestive system is completely bypassed. One of my objectives is to help people with IBD learn how to identify foods and other things that cause flare-ups, so they can eliminate or at least better manage them. Another is to help keep foods that cause flare-ups to a minimum and to reduce the detrimental effects they can have on overall health.

Many people say that diet can't help inflammatory bowel disease. But that notion flies in the face of experience. *Every* chronic illness can be helped by diet. Many chronic illnesses that are subject to flare-up can become dormant or, to be more precise, can go into remission with the help of proper diet. Examples of how diet can help are all around us:

- Diabetics must take insulin every day. They can reduce insulin intake to a minimum if they follow a diet rich in complex carbohydrates and fiber.
- Hypertension—high blood pressure—can be controlled by medication. Hypertensives can also reduce their medication by about 85 percent through diet alone.
- Rheumatoid arthritis and its variations can't be cured, not even by the "right" diet. However, diet can help minimize inflammation and reduce medication—and make life much better.
- Paraplegics can improve the quality of their lives by good dietary management. Inactivity causes them to get bladder infections; a diet that produces high levels of benzoic acid in the urine prevents this. It calls for eating some benzoic acid-producing foods, such as cranberries, or a variation called cloudberries.
- Gout—a buildup of uric acid in the system—can be treated more effectively by diet than by medication. Medication is the treatment of last resort.

Many other examples illustrate how good diet planning can improve the quality of life when you've got a chronic illness. Put it this way: Good diet can't possibly make the illness worse, and it can usually help a great deal. So why not give it a try?

My Interest in Inflammatory Bowel Disease

I hadn't heard about inflammatory bowel disease until about five years ago. Ulcerative colitis, colitis, and Crohn's disease were just words. Then I was invited on a cross-Canada speaking tour. A pretty young woman handled my travel arrangements and accompanied me on this tour. I noticed that she would leave for the lavatory at least once during each meal and sometimes between meals. My curiosity got the best of me; tactfully, I asked her if she was feeling all right. She explained that she had Crohn's disease. This prompted me to ask her more about it.

Then I became more aware of people asking questions following my lectures pertaining to diet and bowel disorder; I started paying more attention to them. I learned that there are many individuals with Crohn's disease, colitis, and ulcerative colitis; they actually number in the millions. The people with this disorder look normal and don't usually talk about it. But once I broke the ice, people with IBD opened up and discussed their disorder. I became interested and decided to learn about the diseases, the people who get them, and what good nutrition can do for them. What developed was very rewarding.

I asked people who have IBD for information about themselves, what foods they eat, and what foods cause IBD to flare up and/or stop an attack. My inquiry started with a few people, grew to about 50, and as of now, I'm corresponding with more than 100 people.

Basics

The Small Intestine

Digestion begins in the mouth. When we chew our food we mix it with saliva, a lubricant that helps to break down starches. Chewing also breaks food into small pieces, increasing its surface area, so the digestive enzymes of the stomach can break it down into protein, fat, carbohydrate, dietary fiber, and a number of vitamins and minerals. (Enzymes are proteins made by our body to carry on our specific functions. The enzymes made by the stomach are for digesting food.) After that, the partially digested food leaves the stomach and enters the intestines. The basic units of protein, fat, carbohydrates, and the vitamins and minerals are absorbed as they pass through the small intestine; and small amounts of these nutrients are absorbed in the stomach.

The *small intestine* is about 20 feet long and is actually three organs. The upper part, the *duodenum*, is where most of the digestion of food actually occurs. Here, thanks to the pancreas, which produces many digestive enzymes and passes them into the duodenum, protein, fat, and carbohydrates are completely broken down into their simplest chemical building blocks. (I'll describe these building blocks in other chapters.) At the same time bile acids, produced in the liver, are passed from the gallbladder through the bile duct into the duodenum. In a way, bile acids are natural human soaps. They combine with fats and help to mix them with water so the enzymes from the pancreas can break them down into simple parts.

The middle section of the small intestine, the *jejunum*, is where the digestion of food and absorption of the building-block chemicals from the food into the blood continue at a maximum. (Absorption into the blood implies that the inside of the digestive system is sort of external to the body. In a way, the digestive system is like a long digestive vat where food is reduced to its simplest chemical subunits so it can enter the blood. In unusual cases, the bowels can be completely bypassed, and the building-block chemicals put directly into the blood.)

After the jejunum comes the *ileum*. Absorption continues to take place in the ileum, but much of the material entering this section is nondigestible residue and will pass from the ileum through a valve into the large intestine, the next part of the bowel. Food spends about four hours going from the mouth to the ileum where, if everything is normal, it's reduced mostly to water, dissolved minerals, and undigested residue called dietary fiber. Passage through the entire small intestine takes from one to two hours. Food is moved along by the muscles in the intestinal wall. These muscles squeeze the food along in wavelike motion called peristalsis.

The Large Intestine

The large intestine consists of four sections: the *ascending colon, transverse colon, descending colon,* and the *sigmoid colon.* Water and minerals are exchanged in the ascending and transverse sections. "Exchanged" means that they are absorbed into the body from the intestinal contents. Under some conditions, water is also released into the intestine and increases the water content of the stool. This passing of water can also include the loss of minerals, such as potassium and calcium.

Microorganisms live in the large intestine; they break down the undigestible residue in food and dietary fiber even more. This natural process produces some important byproducts, and converts the residue to a paste we call the stool. The bacteria actually produce vitamin K in the process. The last section of the intestine, the sigmoid colon, connects to the anus. It is not a simple tube, but consists of a series of valves and baffles that help move the stool along. The anus is actually a valve that connects the digestive system to the external environment.

For those who seek more detailed information on the bowel and its functions, I refer to *Your Gut Feelings*, a book recommended in the Suggested Readings. Your library will also have a selection of books on this subject. Be sure also to use home medical guides and encyclopedias. I strongly recommend reading literature published by the National Foundation for Ileitis and Colitis.

The Bowel Can Be Injured

These seven ingenious organs we collectively call the bowel can be injured. Injury can be due to a bacterial infection, viruses, or other parasites; it can be caused by chemicals that probably get in through food; injury can even come from smoking. Injury can also be due to physical causes, such as exposure to temperature extremes and radiation, or from severe trauma, such as a blow to the abdomen during an accident. Whatever the cause of injury, part or all of the bowel usually becomes inflamed.

A Simplistic View of Inflammation

An inflamed bowel is similar in some respects to other inflamed tissues. You know from experience that inflammation has several characteristics. A joint inflamed by arthritis is swollen, tender, sensitive to touch, sensitive to temperature extremes, doesn't function well, and often can't be relied upon at all. The inflamed tissue hurts when it's resting and even more when you try to use it. Chemicals can relieve the pain, but some chemicals cause it to hurt more. Rest seems to be the best remedy for inflamed tissues, especially those around a joint.

An inflamed bowel is also swollen. Since the bowel is a tubelike organ, swelling causes the opening to get smaller. In fact, the small intestine can swell so much that its central opening is about as small as the circumference of a knitting needle or a piece of string. When an inflamed intestine is used for digestion, it hurts. Remember, peristalsis to the intestine is like bending an ankle or knee. When the intestine is healthy, there's no problem; when it's inflamed, it hurts or doesn't work at all. Like an inflamed joint, an inflamed intestine is sensitive to both chemicals and touch and to some food chemicals, such as spices, or coarse bits and pieces of food, such as fruit or vegetable peels or uneaten nuts.

Additionally, the intestine is lined with a sensitive membrane like that which lines our mouths. You know that you can scrape a coarse object over the skin with no difficulty. But scrape the same object over your mouth or tongue and you've got trouble. Indeed, you can hurt it if you're not careful. This is also true with the inflamed bowel; it can be hurt by coarse, undigested materials.

Emotions and IBD

Comparison of the bowel with other organs stops with the emotions. Our entire digestive system is involved with our emotions. Who hasn't felt a little sick at the stomach during times of extreme stress? We all know people who have gotten so sick that they vomit or get diarrhea and sometimes are bedridden for a day or two. I've seen people get sick while riding on a merry-go-round or seeing a gory picture. That's an obvious influence of a visual signal on the brain and then on the stomach. That doesn't happen with other areas, such as the ankles or knees, unless the person suffers from rheumatoid arthritis; then there's an indirect comparison that we'll discuss later. For now, we must recognize that the bowels respond to emotions, so it follows that emotional upset, which we usually call stress, can make inflamed bowels worse. And if you've got IBD, emotional stress can cause it to flare up.

An Uncontrolled Flare-up

Carol, a close friend, has IBD and recently had a serious flare-up. Her physician hospitalized her immediately for a two-week period of complete rest with intravenous feeding. After two weeks, she returned home and began work a week later. She has a very responsible position and jumped right back into things. Three weeks later, another flare-up occurred, this time much more serious than the previous one. After a week in the hospital, the physicians concluded that the only solution was removal of her ascending and transverse colon. She feels fortunate that she didn't require a colostomy.

Carol's story is not unusual; in fact, it's not as bad as many, because she has retained normal elimination and doesn't face the problem of a colostomy or pouch. Besides, if she'll take more time with her diet, keep her stress level down, and not allow herself to become run down, she'll be fine. As the old fairy tales would conclude: she can live happily ever after.

What Causes IBD?

No one knows for sure, but there are some pretty good theories. The most prevalent theory puts it in the same league with other inflammatory diseases, such as rheumatoid arthritis. Inflammation is actually a type of defense mounted by the body. In this theory, the disease is started by a virus or bacteria and is caused when the immune system mistakenly attacks one or several of its own tissues. In IBD, the intestine is the target, while in rheumatoid arthritis it's the joint tissue.

Support for the inflammatory disease theory also comes from the observation that 25 percent of those with IBD have a blood relative with the disease. Thus, certain people are more susceptible to these reactions from viral attacks. For example, rheumatoid arthritis affects three women for every man in families. People with susceptibility can be identified by sophisticated techniques. Another type of arthritis, ankylosing spondylitis, can be traced to a bacterial infection and affects ten men for every woman.

Strictures

An inflamed bowel can heal; when it does, a stricture remains. I compare a stricture to scar tissue left behind when a serious injury has healed. In the intestine, it's a ring of scar tissue that goes around the intestine and extends for a short distance in each direction.

A stricture can cause trouble, because it's a flaw in an otherwise homogeneous organ. Because it's not as flexible, a stricture can't move with the surrounding tissue, so it "pulls" when the intestine moves. Partially digested food can become stuck in a stricture, leading to a blockage, which can be painful, and in severe cases, require surgery to clear the obstruction.

When a stricture is present, some foods create problems. We'll see that hard pieces of food, such as bits of nuts, seeds of fruit, or even coarse bran from cereal, cause irritation of these strictures.

Emotional Involvement

While experts have ruled out such emotional disturbances as an unhappy childhood or other psychological conditions as causative for IBD, the emotions are clearly involved for its onset and the onset of flare-ups. Here's where the comparison to arthritis makes even more sense. I'll explain.

An IBD Theory

In writing *The Arthritis Relief Diet*, I interviewed hundreds of people with rheumatoid arthritis. In every case there was evidence of a serious viral infection in youth, adolescence, or early adulthood. The virus could have been a severe flu, mononucleosis, or what is now called "chronic fatigue syndrome." It's theorized by experts that after the early infection, the virus lies dormant in the membranes that line the joints.

Some years later, usually between ages 20 and 35, a serious physical or emotional stress occurred and arthritis started. Stress ranged from the trauma of an auto accident or a serious chill, to divorce, damaged relationships, or the death of a loved one. The experts say that the virus starts to multiply and the joint becomes inflamed. In defense, the immune system goes awry and starts attacking the body's own tissues—in rheumatoid arthritis, the tissues that line the joints. If this happens often enough or continuously, the membranes become overgrown and can destroy the joint. The observation that many women get it following childbirth squares with changes in the immune system during pregnancy.

Emotional involvement and stress can be explained in two ways. Severe stress brings about a decline in the immune capacity and the dormant virus starts multiplying. Alternatively, stress creates an imbalance in systems that regulate body functions and inflammation goes unchecked. I speculate that both systems are involved.

Similar to IBD, rheumatoid arthritis, once established, often goes into remission or a phase of remission where medicine is required to keep it "quiet." Further, stress in the form of a change in the weather, a chill, emotional trauma, being overtired, or internal stress created at work or home can cause a flare-up of arthritis. Food can also cause arthritis to flare up; in fact, I have seen one physician inject extracts of beef into arthritis volunteers to demonstrate this point to millions of viewers. Other scientists have reported the food involvement at scientific meetings with less spectacular demonstrations using charts and graphs.

IBD has many similarities to rheumatoid arthritis. Emotional trauma characterizes the sufferers of this illness. Diet too is clearly a factor in two ways: it can trigger a flare-up, and it can cause physical irritation to the bowels. When I question people about food, some can identify, very specifically, foods that cause a flare-up. Many people point to the same foods, such as beets, corn, and chocolate, whereas others seem to react to foods that are a problem only for them, such as slightly unripe bananas.

Several people I spoke with have flare-ups from IBD twice a year—in the fall and spring. The only thing that it can be attributed to is the weather, which changes dramatically in those seasons. Alternatively, seasonal changes place plant and insect irritants, such as pollen, dust, and other materials, in the air, which may result in inflamed sinuses. These sensitivities can also cause IBD to flare up in some people. Seasonal influence has also been researched in rheumatoid arthritis, and there's no doubt of the connection between weather changes and flare-ups. In fact the fall is called "arthritis season" in England.

The fact that IBD can cause symptoms in other parts of the body, such as the eyes, mouth, head, or joints, tells us that it's also a systemic disease. That means that something is produced in one part of the body and is carried by the blood to another part, where it surfaces as a rash or something else. It's tempting to think that the bowel produces materials that can be picked up in the blood. In fact, it's an avenue of active research that has yielded some positive results. These scientific discoveries make IBD look more and more like a type of rheumatoid arthritis or vice versa. Not surprisingly, many people with IBD are treated by rheumatologists.

Who Gets IBD?

Anyone can get IBD. There's no sex differentiation; women and men seem to get it with equal rates. The greatest number who get it are between the ages of 12 and 40. About 10 percent are under age 12. It seems to run in families in about 25 percent of the cases. It's not clear whether that correlation is caused by heredity or environment. Only serious research will uncover this aspect of the disease.

Psychology

There does seem to be a psychological profile for people with IBD. Most people I interviewed had difficulty dealing with emotions in childhood, and many had had an unsettling family life. In short, their lives were characterized by emotional upset. However, I've also talked to many IBD sufferers who are stable, joyful, and come from happy homes. This leads me to believe that the connection is how they deal with stress.

Many people with IBD just plain don't deal well with

stress. They say, "I just keep my mouth shut," or "There was no one to talk it out with." Even though this doesn't show cause and effect, it does indicate that the body responds to stress in various ways. Some people with IBD describe themselves as "professional internalizers." And although that's not a fair description of even a significant number of IBD sufferers, it does seem to describe some.

One doctor who practices at a major university gave me an interesting insight. His comment was, "Exam time is Crohn's time. Most of our diagnoses are made during examination time. That's when the kids are under stress and stress brings it out every time!" Another doctor showed me two letters. He said, "I can always identify the IBD patient." One letter I received was written without respect for margins; the writing was small, and it went from edge to edge. Every square inch of paper was used. The other was quite normal. He said, "I can always spot the people with intestinal disorders when they write me a letter. They're usually a variation of this."

Although I don't feel that IBD is the direct result of any psychological cause and effect, I do believe that the emotions have a major effect on the emergence and course of the disease. When I asked what caused flare-ups, every person with IBD mentioned variations on two things: stress and food.

People often describe fatigue as a cause of flare-ups. Fatigue is a fuzzy description, because it may mean that someone is tired from overwork or from exercising too much, or tired from not enough rest or sleep. It can also come from poor nutrition. Since so many people say that fatigue, stress, and food are the major culprits in flare-ups, I have come to believe they are all interinvolved. In Chapter Twenty-two, we explore the help an IBD patient can get from a support group. Some groups use professionally trained discussion leaders to help people explore their emotions. By discussing your emotions openly, you learn to deal with stress. You'll find that there's a solution to every problem.

Medical Treatment

IBD is usually treated first with some dietary modification. In general, this approach is summarized in a few sentences: Don't eat Chinese food; peel all fruit; boil vegetables to soften them, and so on. Next, or concurrently, comes medication—steroids to stop flare-ups, Azulfadine to reduce inflammation, and sometimes tranquilizers to calm the emotions.

Once medication has been used and a major flare-up occurs, the only solution left is surgery. Surgery usually means a removal of part of the intestine and often an artificial opening in the abdomen—an "ostomy" of some type. With this sequence of events as a backdrop, I urge you to use diet and food as much as possible to reduce inflammation and prevent flare-ups.

Diet and Self-Health Management

Good nutrition is essential to good health. I agree with the experts: diet can't cure IBD, but without good health practices, IBD will drag you down and you may never be able to recover. With good nutrition, the correct food, and personal stress management, you can reduce the flare-ups to a minimum. I call that "optimum health." It's the state of health where you're doing the best for yourself. That's "self-health management" and it begins with good nutrition.

PART ONE

Meeting Nutritional
Challenges

Like any other chronic disease, IBD creates some special nutritional challenges. These include identifying foods that aggravate or cause flare-ups, but also foods that help make a flare-up subside. You can identify these foods by a number of well-tested methods, including keeping a food diary.

Other challenges include meeting the need for the correct dietary fiber and choosing food supplements that deliver everything they should. There may be times when a vitamin pill isn't enough and special supplement foods are necessary. These special medicinal foods provide complete nutrition with a minimum amount of work by the bowels. Supplements can also be used to overcome lactose intolerance and the need for soluble dietary fiber.

Each of these and other issues are dealt with in the next nine chapters. Some challenges can be met easily and clearly; others have only general solutions to help people with IBD manage their illness more effectively. This enhances the effectiveness of the physician's management of the disease.

By applying every effort possible, the quality of life will improve. It'll be possible to "smell the roses" more acutely.

CHAPTER ONE

Nutritional Challenges
for People with IBD

From the mildest cold virus to the most devastating cancer, illness increases the need for vitamins and minerals and changes the need to distribute calories between fat, protein, and carbohydrate. Illness also changes the amount and type of dietary fiber needed. Inflammatory bowel disease, in particular, imposes serious nutritional challenges that must be dealt with daily and especially during flare-ups.

Malabsorption of Vitamins and Minerals

Inflamed tissue doesn't function as well as it should; you know something's wrong because it hurts. Accordingly, an inflamed intestine does not function as well as it should. Absorption of nutrients is impaired and some nutrients are actually lost—that is, not absorbed. Malabsorption literally means "sick absorption."

Malabsorption of vitamins and minerals is variable and

depends on where the small intestine is inflamed. Most vitamins and many minerals are absorbed throughout the small intestine, and some vitamins are even absorbed from the stomach. Vitamin B_{12} is absorbed only in the lower 4 feet of the small intestine and depends on the secretion of a factor from the stomach. Therefore, if the most severely inflamed portion is the terminal 4 feet, or if it's been removed, B_{12} absorption is impaired or nonexistent. Some minerals, such as zinc, are absorbed from the large intestine; if that's damaged or removed, it presents another problem. The other vitamins and minerals can be dealt with by the process chemists call "mass action" and nutritionists call "supplementation."

I use the term *mass action*, because in malabsorption the percentage of nutrients normally absorbed is reduced. We overcome that problem by making more nutrients available. For example, if 25 percent of magnesium is absorbed from a normal bowel, but because of inflammation or surgery only 50 percent of normal absorption is possible, then only 12 or 13 percent of dietary magnesium will be absorbed. Therefore, we should strive to get not 400 milligrams per day, but 800 milligrams per day. The only way is through good food choice and the sensible use of food supplements. I emphasize "sensible" because you can't take just any vitamin pill and expect it to solve the problem. I've devoted Chapter Seven to supplement selection.

Vitamin K presents a special case. We rely on food for part of our vitamin K need and on intestinal microbes for the rest. Impaired absorption is likely to reduce the vitamin K absorbed from food. And with other intestinal problems, such as diarrhea, or removal of some of the intestine, we're likely not to get enough vitamin K—perhaps none—from our intestinal flora. This deficiency might cause bruises or excessive bleeding from cuts or scrapes. However, the deficiency may not show up until something serious happens. That's why it's important to raise the issue with your physician. A supplement can be prescribed to correct the problem.

Consequences of Malabsorption

Malabsorption can cause malnutrition. Using the meaning of both words, poor absorption can cause poor nutrition. This needn't cause you to despair, because there are reserves available to meet the challenges. These reserves come in the form of food and food supplements. Because the consequence of poor nutrition is poor health, you may need them.

Failure to thrive—a nice way of saying the child has fallen behind in growth and development and lacks energy—is often seen in children with IBD. It's the same problem that's seen in children living in third-world countries where there isn't enough good food to go around. In our children, it means they may be eating well, but the nutrients aren't getting absorbed. They simply aren't getting enough calories and are specifically falling short in protein, vitamins, and minerals.

Similar problems are seen in adults, but since they aren't growing any longer, such problems show up as muscle wasting, inability to gain weight, and a general lack of energy. The adult is absorbing enough calories from food to just get by. Under these conditions women often don't maintain enough body fat and they stop menstruating. This same problem can arise from a lack of protein. Whatever the cause, the only solution is to get more protein-rich foods and calories from carbohydrate-rich foods.

Other consequences of long-term malabsorption include all the nightmarish illnesses of vitamin mineral deficiency. In the beginning these show up as minor problems. Irritability and depression come first, but the most common, overt symptom is cracking of the lips at the corners of the mouth, poor luster of hair, weak, brittle fingernails, chills or feeling cold easily, a lack of energy, and recurring headaches. Do these symptoms sound vague? Do they sound familiar?

Don't we *all* experience these vague symptoms from time to time? Of course we do! But if you have IBD and any of these symptoms persist for days, you'd better see your doctor. The best insurance is to use nutritional supplements so the symptoms aren't from poor nutrition. Supplements come in many forms and can ensure good nutrition.

I've summarized the symptoms of deficiency in Table 1.1. As you look at this table, you may see very quickly that you've had every symptom. I can assure you that I have also, because they come from lots of minor illnesses, including minor stress from work, just plain being overtired, or a coming cold. When the symptoms persist, you should do something; that includes eating properly, taking food supplements, and having a discussion with your doctor. However, the best medicine is prevention in the form of good nutrition.

Special Challenges of Macronutrients

Fat, protein, and carbohydrate create other challenges. You can't take a supplement to make up for them. They require careful planning for several reasons; you probably require more protein than average because of malabsorption, increased loss, and increased basal metabolism; you must reduce fat to eliminate the cramps and diarrhea that result from poor absorption; and you've got to get more calories from carbohydrate to make up for a decrease in fat. This calls for nutritional teamwork.

This challenge can be overcome in several ways. The first is to eat high-protein, low-fat, easily digested meats. This translates to fish, fowl, easily digested red meats, such as ground lean beef, and eggs. Second is to get enough calories. That means more complex cabohydrates from foods that don't irritate the bowels, such as rice, potatoes, and pasta. You can use milk and other dairy products to advantage, especially yogurt and certain kinds of cheese.

One means of meeting the protein need is simply to use a supplemental food. Products are available that can provide a nice tasty "shake" that's high in protein, contains little or no fat, moderate carbohydrate, and is high in calories.

Diarrhea and Nutrition

Diarrhea causes a loss of nutrients. This loss is especially important with the electrolytes—the salts needed by your body to maintain correct fluid balance, nervous system function, and general health. The electrolytes consist mostly of sodium, potassium, and chloride. We'll discuss them in much more detail in Chapter Twenty-one. Electrolytes, especially potassium, are critical, because potassium isn't easily taken as a supplement. For now, recognize that diarrhea requires special attention to diet.

Diarrhea results from an inability of the intestine to deal with bile acids. Bile acids are produced in the liver and passed into the upper end of the small intestine, where they help fat be digested. Bile acids are reabsorbed in the lower small intestine. Because the small intestine is often impaired in IBD, the bile acids get passed into the large intestine, where they cause watery diarrhea. Lack of reabsorption of bile acids causes a loss of the bile acids and that leads to poor fat absorption; poor fat absorption produces especially foul stools and watery diarrhea. There are two solutions: Reduce fat intake and increase the correct type of dietary fiber. (Correct dietary fiber means soluble fiber from oatmeal, not hard fiber from wheat bran. See pages 65 and 207.) It can also mean a soluble fiber supplement, such as Metamucil, to help firm up the stools and absorb the bile acids.

Medication and Nutrition

Every medication known increases nutritional requirements; no medication has ever been developed that decreases nutritional requirements! When I'm a guest speaker, I like to ask my audience how many people have used aspirin or a version of aspirin; usually most hands go up. Then, how many of them have given baby aspirin to their children; most hands go up. Finally, the big question: "How many of you include some extra vitamin C and B vitamins with the aspirin, especially if you use aspirin more than once?" I get a lot of blank stares!

These days no one gets scurvy because they take aspirin. Our diet is usually sufficient in vitamin C and B vitamins to compensate for the loss. But what about people who take 12 aspirins daily for arthritis pain? If they don't eat a well-balanced diet, with special attention to these nutrients, they could easily fall short. I'm sure they won't get scurvy, which is the end result of a long deficiency and not the result of a marginal deficiency. However, I'm sure most people would feel better if they took a vitamin C and a B-complex supplement, or even better, ate an extra orange or two during the day and an extra serving of meat or fish for the B vitamins.

Medications used for IBD range from the corticosteroids that increase the need for the B-complex of vitamins, to the resin cholestyramine that can reduce the absorption of important minerals and the water-soluble vitamins. Corticosteroids and Azulfidine are used to quiet flare-ups and stop inflammation. Cholestyramine (Questran) firms the stools and stops diarrhea by absorbing bile acids. Unfortunately, the nutritional effects of prescription drugs are seldom discussed. Therefore, very little specific information is available. Some general observations are helpful, however.

Because food often interferes with the absorption of medication and medication interferes with the absorption of nutrients, some medication should be taken between meals. Your doctor might not know exactly how they should be taken, but the pharmacist should; so make sure you ask. Persist until you get a definite answer. Alternatively, either purchase a book like *The People's Pharmacy*, or go to the library and look up the drug you've been prescribed in the *Physician's Desk Reference of Prescription Drugs* (see Suggested Reading). These books contain information about the known nutritional interactions. They won't be able to explain the increased nutritional need that results from the drug, but they will identify side effects, such as "dizziness" or "dry mouth."

Prolonged use of any prescription medication usually results in gradual nutrient depletion. For example, aspirin depletes vitamin C and the constant loss of blood caused by aspirin leads to anemia; antibiotics inhibit absorption of iron and sometimes calcium. To make matters worse, no research has been done on the nutritional effects of drugs taken in combination. My correspondence with IBD patients indicates that many take four or more different medications daily. Each of these medications exerts a profound physiological effect or it wouldn't have been prescribed. What about when they're used in combination? We know that they increase nutritional needs, but we don't know to what extent. And no one knows the total effect when so many medications are taken in combination.

There are several things the IBD sufferer can do. Make sure your diet is as good as it can be. Support a good diet with sensible nutritional supplements to be sure your body has all the nutrients it requires. Consult with your physician and pharmacist and use library resources to learn as much as possible about the effects of your medication. Talk about medication at support group meetings to learn everything you can about their side effects.

Stress

Any chronic illness is stressful. IBD seems to be stress related in both its origins and the onset of flare-ups. It follows that stress is part of the life of an IBD sufferer. And stress has been shown to increase nutritional requirements. This has been studied on normal people under stress and is especially true of people with a chronic illness.

With IBD you *must* avoid and manage stress. We'll talk about stress management in Chapter Twenty-two. But keep in mind that there is a nutritional component to stress; diet can help to increase or moderate the effects. For example, when we eat food that's high in sugar or salt, we're stressing our body's metabolism. Excessive dietary sugar first increases, then decreases blood sugar; this influences our emotions and creates anxiety. A similar situation arises with excessive alcohol, although alcoholic beverages are generally avoided by folks with IBD. We also increase our stress level by eating foods that cause IBD flare-ups.

Stress management with diet requires that we seek foods that do not contain empty calories from sugar or fat. Similarly, we cause our body to overwork when we eat foods with excessive sodium and not enough potassium. That's stress! Strive for foods containing complex carbohydrates and nonirritating, soluble fiber. (See Chapter Thirteen.) Eat a diet that will not provoke flare-ups. Seek foods that have a good K factor (are rich in potassium). Strive to get sufficient protein from low-fat sources; if necessary, use protein supplements. Be sure to get adequate amounts of vitamins and minerals; if in doubt, get a safe excess of all nutrients as a form of nutritional insurance.

Caffeine

About 10,000 years ago, tea was discovered in China; coffee came much later. Each beverage supplies the same stimulant—caffeine. A typical cup of tea contains about 35 milligrams of caffeine; the same as a 12-ounce can of cola. A cup of coffee delivers from 100 to 150 milligrams of caffeine, depending on how it's brewed. Strong coffee is traditional with many people, and caffeine is responsible for the "lift" that we get from it.

Caffeine is one of a group of physiologically active and addictive chemicals called alkaloids. In other words, caffeine is a drug that stimulates the central nervous system. It gives you a lift as do many other drugs; it's just that the lift from caffeine isn't generally harmful or as intense as it is from other drugs. It's just as addictive, however—as addictive as harmful drugs like cocaine, heroin, and nicotine. Indeed, when people who drink large amounts of coffee stop using coffee, they usually experience the same withdrawal symptoms as those from drugs, including anxiety, irritability, paranoia, and even sickness. The symptoms are just not as dramatic as withdrawal from street drugs.

Caffeine lifts you up and when the caffeine is gone from your body, it lets you down. You'll feel more tired and seem to have less energy. Both experiences have an effect on nutrition.

Caffeine increases the need for calcium. For reasons that aren't completely clear, heavy coffee drinkers have increased incidence of osteoporosis. They excrete more calcium than noncoffee or tea drinkers. Don't rely on a little milk or cream in coffee to make up for the loss; you'd better count on a glass of milk, 8 ounces of yogurt, or a calcium supplement.

Serious Flare-ups

Serious flare-ups often cause physicians to take a dramatic step—prescribing a complete liquid formula diet. This diet usually consists of a formula food that comes in a can or a bottle. If your flare-up is not too serious, your doctor may prescribe a food made up from a powder which contains no fiber or anything that's undigestible. Such foods are completely absorbed; we call these formulas "low residue." The objective is to give your digestive system a complete rest. And it works! After a couple of weeks on these liquid products, you can slowly start eating foods, beginning with broth and working up slowly to easily digested carbohydrates and meats.

Think of it this way. Suppose you twist your ankle. The doctor might tape it and say, "Stay completely off it for a week; then, you can slowly start with a wheelchair, progress to crutches, and finally walk carefully." Your intestine is no different; it's just that you rest your intestine by putting nothing in it.

TPN:
Total Parenteral Nutrition

Use of total parenteral nutrition (TPN) started many years ago with people who were severely injured. These people didn't have enough small intestine left to get any nutrition. The only hope was to put nourishment into them through a large vein. The process works and, thanks to dedicated researchers, is now a routine procedure.

There are people alive today who haven't eaten in years. These people come home from a normal day's work and hook themselves up to a machine that pumps the elements of food into their body. It's the only way they can stay alive. And they don't just survive, they thrive! TPN is a high-tech answer to a problem that was once deadly—the ultimate marriage between nutrition and technology. Nutrients bypass the digestive system completely. People who must survive by this means can lead a normal, productive, and abundant life.

TPN is also employed to give the small intestine a complete short-term rest. Think over the twisted-ankle analogy. If the small intestine is in trouble, why not take the same approach? Give it a rest; let it heal. TPN is the solution your physician might choose.

If you ever need TPN, you'll be in the hands of a sophisticated team. The team led by the physician includes dieticians, nurses, medical technologists, and sociologists. They'll work together with the objective of restoring health to your digestive system and get you back on real food.

The symptoms listed in Table 1.1 are often observed when people are marginally deficient in the nutrient mentioned. However, they are also associated with other more or less serious illnesses, complications of illness, or the side effects of medication. If any of them persist, be sure your diet and dietary supplements are correct, and see your physician.

TABLE 1.1
Common Symptoms of Minor Nutrient Deficiencies

Symptom	Nutritional Deficit
Failure to thrive Poor growth in children Tiredness in adults Muscle wasting	Insufficient calories, protein, and some micronutrients
Cold feeling, poor complexion, tiredness	Anemia, especially of iron and folic acid
Sore mouth, cracks at corners of lips, sore tongue	B complex of vitamins, especially folic acid
Loss of taste and smell Cuts don't heal quickly Post-adolescent acne	Zinc deficiency
Mild depression Confusion, irritability	B-complex deficiency, especially folic acid
Muscle aches Low back pain	Calcium-magnesium deficiency
Muscle weakness, spasm Numbness and tingling	Electrolytes, especially potassium and possibly sodium
Bruises, cuts don't heal quickly	Vitamin K and possibly vitamin C

CHAPTER TWO

What People Tell Me: Putting Thoughts into Food

We'll discuss the basics of nutrition in Part Two, but we don't eat nutrients, we eat food. Therefore, we've got to avoid foods that cause flare-ups, discomfort, and diarrhea. Remember, each person is an individual, and food that's all right for one person is not always okay for another. Some foods seem to be generally unacceptable for everyone with IBD; I'll try to help you avoid these foods. More important, I'll emphasize foods that seem to agree with most people.

Flare-ups: Diarrhea

It's difficult to separate a flare-up from diarrhea, so I'll define a few terms. A flare-up usually includes serious pain. Marc said it well: "It starts as a pain around my navel and progresses throughout my abdomen. Then the diarrhea comes." Marc rests for a day or so without eating and the flare-up goes away. That's not always the case, however.

Some people have such serious flare-ups and intense pain that they must be hospitalized. When this happens, complete rest of the bowel is accomplished by intravenous feeding or by using a predigested food supplement. In very serious flare-ups nutrition is achieved by providing all nourishment through a large vein; this is called TPN, short for Total Parenteral Nutrition. The last resort is surgery.

Surgery often involves removal of part of the bowel; it is usually confined to a section of the large intestine. In many cases, the patient is left with a temporary or permanent ostomy. An ostomy is an opening in the abdomen, which allows stools to pass into a bag that you attach and remove yourself. The surgeon can often build an internal pouch that acts as a reservoir, in which the waste collects. The pouch is regularly emptied into an appliance. Surgeons have other variations on these procedures to make life as normal as possible after surgery.

Many people point out that the surgery brings relief. Indeed, they go further and say that it has at least allowed them to live a normal life. Before surgery, any trip to the store or to visit a friend might end in a dash home because of painful cramps and diarrhea. People even plan vacations around the IBD. Even after surgery, however, many people continue to experience flare-ups. For them the specter of more surgery hangs heavy. They, too, must practice prevention of flare-ups.

Foods can cause flare-ups and diarrhea. In some cases the flare-up follows immediately. As Mrs. Arthur O. put it, "I suspected beet juice as the culprit so I drank some. Within thirty minutes it was expelled in my watery stool!" She goes on to explain that for her beet juice is like a diabolical poison. "I'd rather starve than drink it. I can't describe how devastating it is to me!" Actually there's a slight misconception here; you couldn't eat something and have it pass in 30 minutes. In this case beets are so irritating to Mrs. O. that they precipitate a violent reaction, possibly including the passage of some blood.

In contrast to Mrs. Arthur O., a few people claim they

can eat just about anything. They have only flare-ups twice yearly. They seem to be in the minority. There's no doubt that their IBD is not triggered by food, but by something in the air. (On the other hand, not a single person could tolerate stress and fatigue. We'll cover that in Chapter Twenty-two.)

At times some people can eat almost anything. I think it's best said by Janet. "When I'm in remission, like I am now, I can eat anything I want; but not large quantities or I get very full and want to vomit. One day I would eat pizza or tacos or yogurt and be fine and the very next day I could eat the exact same things and be sick for two days."

Foods that Cause Flare-ups and Diarrhea

I asked people to identify foods that constantly cause flare-ups for them. Some people claim that no foods cause flare-ups. They argue the flare-up is caused by stress. Eileen said it quite clearly. "Stress causes the flare-ups. Certain foods *aggravate* flare-ups, but none *cause* it."

A word of caution. This information is not scientific, but rather anecdotal, meaning the information is the experience of a person, not the findings of research. I doubt that this information can ever be put on a solid scientific footing because it would require serious, very expensive research. We'd have to identify suspect foods and then have people eat them in a predetermined sequence. Obviously, some people would get very sick in the process. To make matters worse, some people would require special medication for the flare-up, some hospitalization, and maybe even surgery. It's not worth it.

An alternative to the research that will never get done is for you to keep an accurate food diary as described in Chapter Three. In this way, you'll be in close touch with your body and will identify the foods that trigger or, as Eileen says, "aggravate" flare-ups. The information here will help to guide you; but remember, it's only a guide. Just because you get some diarrhea from a food, doesn't mean that that specific food is the culprit. You've got to try the food several more times, under different conditions, to be sure. There are very few certainties here.

Table 2.1 lists foods that seem consistently to cause (or aggravate) flare-ups, discomfort, and diarrhea. These foods probably don't tell the entire story. Other patterns have emerged that make me suspect some foods, food additives, and methods of food preparation. I've summarized these in Table 2.2 You should approach these foods and cooking techniques with suspicion and see for yourself. There are no set rules.

Tables 2.1 and 2.2 don't tell the entire story. For example some people can't eat foods that contain MSG (monosodium glutamate). I heard about it only from people who tried it and found out for themselves. Some people ate apples and they caused discomfort, so they stopped eating them. Others peeled the apples and found they were just fine. Similarly for peaches, pears, grapes, and plums.

That's why I've included this chapter. I'm interested in telling you what foods seem to be okay. These are responses to the question: "What foods never cause flare-ups?" I went further in my questioning and asked people to identify specific meats, cereals, and other foods they could always eat.

Foods that *Don't* Cause Flare-ups

Let's be positive and focus on foods that *can* be eaten! I've tried to separate the foods into familiar groups that seem to make life better for folks with IBD. That's what led me to prepare the following listing.

These foods are the ones that *most* people could eat with no discomfort. I emphasize *most* because not everyone who replied could eat them all. Some people eat almost any food in moderation. This listing shows that there are many foods to choose from. I've listed them by category and noted any pertinent facts about preparation.

Cereal: Oatmeal, Cream of Wheat, corn flakes, Bran Flakes, Malt O Meal, Special K, Product 19, and Cheerios. There's a clear avoidance of hard fiber ("fiber matrix") wheat cereals. Many people use milk sparingly.

Dairy Products: Lactaid milk, low-fat and nonfat (skim) milk, yogurt, aged cheese, cottage, and soft cheese.

Eggs: Some people avoided eggs. Those who eat eggs emphasized poached, soft boiled, and hard boiled. Not one respondent could eat fried eggs.

Beef: Lean beef either as roast, steak, or ground and broiled or roasted. No frying. Some people could eat barbecued meat, but were careful to avoid any charring of the meat.

Other Meat: Lean ham, carefully trimmed pork, trimmed lamb and veal. Emphasis was always put on "lean" and "trimmed."

Fish: Fish is universally accepted. I emphasize fish that swim; they're called finfish. They include tuna, swordfish, salmon, halibut, fillets of flounder and other fish, snapper and most other finfish. Those who tried it could eat it. Preparation includes broiling, poaching, or baking. No one ate fried fish!

Shellfish: Scallops are all right if broiled or poached. Many people emphasized that they couldn't eat shellfish, such as clams and oysters, or crustaceans, including lobster and crab.

Poultry: Everyone who responded could eat white meat of poultry with two provisos: the skin must be removed and the meat cannot be fried and breaded. Some people need to avoid dark poultry meat. Roasted, broiled, barbecued poultry is fine, but never fried.

Vegetables: With the wide variety of vegetables, I've tried to group them into categories most people are familiar with.

Potatoes: Potatoes are always eaten without the skin. Eat them baked, boiled, or mashed. Sweet potatoes and yams are fine if well cooked and peeled.

Skin Vegetables: Carrots, squash, tomatoes, cucum-

bers, celery, jicama. The skin must be removed. Most
respondents said that they had to cook these vegetables
until they were soft.

Vegetables with Skin: Broccoli, cauliflower, brussels
sprouts, asparagus, all string beans, and peas. These vegetables must be cooked well by boiling. Steaming is acceptable for some folks, but the vegetables must be
steamed until soft.

Beans: Some beans can simply be boiled; these include limas, navy beans, chick-peas, and lentils. Other
beans, such as black, pinto, kidney, red beans, or gar-
banzos, must be cooked almost to a mush. Some people
can eat canned baked beans.

Leafy Vegetables: Lettuce is fine for everyone. Spinach is all right for most people when boiled well. Cabbage, if well cooked, is acceptable to a few people, but
most insist they must avoid it at all costs.

Fruit: Emphasis should be placed on peeling. It seems
that most fruit is acceptable if it's been peeled. Apples,
pears, peaches (when peeled), avocados, bananas (if not
green), apricots (if fully ripe and peeled), plums (if fully
ripe and peeled), strawberries and kiwifruit, canned
peaches, plums, pears, apples, etc., oranges and grapefruit. (Carefully avoid the fibrous section in grapefruit.)

Grains: Boiled white and brown rice, pasta, egg noo-
dles, macaroni. Breads and rolls without seeds, including
white, rye, wheat, five-grain, French, and Italian bread.
Absolutely no seed of any type—sesame, poppy, etc.

Processed Foods: Most respondents avoided processed
foods, but there are many that others use: canned fruit,
canned applesauce, baked beans for some people. A
surprising number eat pretzels, bagels and some cookies.
No chocolate chips!

Beverages: Most people could use fruit juices, and
vegetable juices, such as tomato and V-8 juice. Specific
fruit juices were orange, grapefruit, cranberry, and apple. Tea, iced and hot, not strong; caffeine-free cola and
other carbonated beverages; mineral water, distilled wa-

ter, and reverse-osmosis purified water; ginger ale, 7-Up, limeade, herb tea, soy milk; coffee and alcohol very sparingly.

What I've Learned from the Eating Patterns

Irritation of the intestinal tract must be avoided. By trial and error, guidance from physicians, and talking to other people, IBD sufferers seem to learn what's okay for them. It helps to keep a careful food diary. There are some basics that apply to everyone.

Small portions and frequent meals seem to be a universal pattern. Indeed, my impression is that if portions and meals are kept small, a wider variety of food is acceptable. That's logical because the intestine doesn't need to deal with a large quantity of any single material, and a small meal is likely to be well chewed. And there are portion thresholds for most foods that cause or aggravate flare-ups.

Another point was made very clear by Mrs. Arthur O. "Chew, chew, chew your food!" She and most other people emphasized small, well-chewed portions of food. This advice is probably the most practical of all that will help everyone. I can't emphasize it enough. CHEW FOOD THOROUGHLY.

Fatty foods are bad news. Some fat can be tolerated, however, if it's taken along with a starch. For example, a small piece of lean roast beef, baked potato, and cooked green vegetables are all right. But putting gravy on the potatoes or the roast beef spells trouble.

Some fiber is necessary and helpful. For example, oatmeal, Cream of Wheat, bananas, and most peeled fruit are excellent. That tells me that a fiber matrix, or in more scientific terms, the intact cellulose matrix in plant foods such as a fruit peel or hard bean, especially wheat bran, is out. This pattern is very good. It means that some cereals, especially those with soluble fiber, such as oatmeal, are ideal and that fiber supplements are beneficial.

Most people emphasized well-cooked vegetables; for example, mushy beans or asparagus. This verifies the need to break down the fiber matrix. Once these foods are thoroughly cooked, they are okay. One pitfall of this is the definite loss of some vitamins and potassium by this extensive cooking.

Most people with IBD avoid caffeine, food additives, and spices. People with IBD are especially sensitive to spices, stimulants, and food chemicals, including MSG, saccharine, and others. Again, emphasize the need for a food diary and natural foods. Special attention must always be paid to cooking methods.

Universal avoidance of frying and of large portions of fatty meats highlights the difficulty with fat. It is probably more than the fat in these meats that causes the problem. Fat is often associated with tough membranes; these could be irritating to the intestinal wall in a manner similar to an apple peel. Nonetheless, fat itself is definitely a problem. Difficulty with fat is also obvious by the wide acceptance of white meat, rather than dark, from poultry and fish. A low-fat diet is naturally best for folks with IBD. It allows them to live in harmony with nature and stay in better health generally.

These observations made me curious about food as a therapeutic aid, so I asked another question, "Are there any foods that stop flare-ups or diarrhea?" I was pleasantly surprised.

Foods that Help Stop Flare-ups and Diarrhea

EILEEN: "If there was a single food to stop the flare-ups I'd be at the grocery store and not the hospital." Eileen was writing to me from the hospital bed!

Although most people simply stop eating, rest, and take medication, others have experimented to find helpful foods to take along with these other measures. A few observations emerge.

Supplemental foods can help reset the bowels, while giving complete nutrition. I discuss these in Chapter Eight. Criticare HN by Bristol-Meyers and Vital by Ross Labs come as close to complete digestive rest as possible. What makes me so enthusiastic about these products is their excellent nutritional support and ability to rest the digestive system. When IBD patients don't eat, they run a serious risk due to loss of electrolytes (see Chapter Twenty-one) and other nutrients. Criticare and Vital prevent nutrient deficiency and bring them "through the storm" while resting the system.

Soft soluble fiber in the form of Metamucil, Daily Fiber Blend, or some other brand, help to stop the diarrhea. Some people use them on a daily basis. Others use Metamucil only when diarrhea is bad. Creamy oatmeal made by slow cooking and Cream of Wheat seem to help others. Some folks eat ripe bananas and a few eat mashed potatoes or well-cooked brown rice—remedies are based on personal experimentation.

An old folk remedy for diarrhea recommends eating an apple, banana, and cottage cheese. The apple and banana supply soluble fiber, and calcium from the cheese adds more binding capacity. The combination also helps restore the electrolyte balance. The apple must be peeled, of course. These patterns fit with the observation that soft, soluble fiber helps to bind the stools. The original research done on fiber included people with the "diarrhea disease." These folks have chronic diarrhea even though it has not been officially diagnosed as IBD. The original research papers proved that adding fiber to their food stopped the diarrhea.

Fiber firms up the stools by binding water, bile acids, and intestinal irritants. People who deliberately use fiber supplements, such as Metamucil, Daily Fiber Blend, or another fiber supplement, get the best results. It's worth trying in small quantities, at first, and then working up to the regular dose. A few people pointed out that they used clear broth—some even made chicken soup the old-fashioned way—to help. Broth provides electrolytes with a high K factor—or intake of dietary potassium—important because electrolyte loss, especially potassium loss, can cause diarrhea all by itself. More important, electrolyte loss will make people with diarrhea feel sicker than they already do.

I asked people some specific questions about fruit, vegetable, and cereal use. From this I learned that most of them don't get nearly enough fiber. Actually, this is confirmed by other research done in Europe on people with IBD. Those who get the most fiber eat oatmeal, fruit, potatoes, brown rice, and vegetables without skin. There's no proof that this diet makes them feel better, but a small amount of research indicates that it helps them.

Few of the "bran" or whole-grain cereals provide sufficient fiber. And it's important to note that the fiber they provide—cellulose—could be too irritating for the people with IBD. Thus, caution is essential in selecting cereals. In the next chapter we'll review the best cereals to provide dietary fiber.

Vitamin-Mineral Supplements

Many people use food supplements that are prescribed by their doctor. Others require B_{12} injections, largely in the aftermath of surgery. Most supplements provide a good balance of vitamins and minerals, but do not compensate for potassium, fiber, or protein; these nutrients are covered in other chapters.

Hanna put it very clearly; I'll let her speak:

> I started taking supplements in 1983. I've progressively improved since then. Through good nutrition, I have built up my body to a point where my Crohn's disease is not as severe as in the past. I have small flare-ups now as

compared to chronic, life-threatening episodes where I would be hospitalized. My health improved so much that I didn't think twice about becoming pregnant in 1985.

I was surprised at how sensibly people selected their food supplements. In addition to a multivitamin-multimineral supplement, people selected supplements to meet their individual needs. They used calcium, calcium and magnesium, iron, zinc, B complex, vitamins C, E, and beta carotene. The people who use supplements seem to have a more positive attitude and require less medication.

Medications

Medication use by people with IBD is overwhelming. Some people take as many as 20 tablets and capsules of medication daily, not counting vitamin supplements. I've listed most of the medications people take to give you an idea of the variety and scope. You can see that they aren't all being used for IBD; the list contains medications for asthma, anxiety, insomnia, motion sickness, high blood pressure, antipsychotics, and one or two potassium supplements.

I can't help but wonder what additional nutritional requirements these drugs impose on the body. A multivitamin-multimineral supplement is essential at the very least to counteract the stress the drugs cause. Additionally, extra calcium, iron, and zinc are probably appropriate.

Azulfidine (sulfasalazine)	Prednisone
Bumex	Desyrel
Capoten	Seldane
Cardizem	Norpace
Chlorihalidone	Lasix
Corgard	Boataria
Halcion	Elavil
Imodium	Bentyl
K-lite	Lomotil

Lomotil
Parafon Forte
Premarin
Questran
Restoril
Serax
Tagamet
Theo-Dur
Tranxene
Xanax

Medrol
Darvocet-N
Provera
Bentyl
Compazine
Dyazide
Flagyl
Thyroid medication
Zyloprim
ACTH
Elavil

Supplements and Medication

Most medication increases the need for nutrients, and some medication prevents the absorption of nutrients. For example, Questran reduces absorption of some minerals, such as calcium, magnesium, and zinc, as well as some water-soluble vitamins; Azulfidine interferes with folic acid, a B vitamin that's critical to health; simple aspirin causes vitamin-C destruction; and steroids cause calcium, magnesium, and potassium loss and increase sodium retention, which can trigger an increase in blood pressure that requires other medication.

The question from all this is: What's a person to do? The answer: Take a complete, balanced, food-supplement daily, together with specific vitamins and minerals that are especially vulnerable (these include folic acid, calcium, magnesium, zinc, and vitamin C).

Summary

IBD need not restrict the diet unduly. A wide variety of safe foods are available, so folks with IBD can thrive. Care in food preparation is required to avoid flare-ups. Some food can be used to help reduce diarrhea and help make flare-ups less severe. Food supplements make proper nutrition easier and provide complete nourishment. Fried, spicy, and high-fat foods should be avoided. Several small meals are more beneficial than large meals. It's important to chew food thoroughly.

Fiber can be used in supplement form to help control diarrhea. It can also be supportive during remission to help produce good stool consistency. A physician should be consulted to select a nonirritating fiber supplement. Vitamin-mineral supplements can be used effectively to support the diet and insure good nutrition. The widespread use of prescription drugs makes these supplements even more important.

TABLE 2.1
Foods that Cause Flare-ups and Diarrhea

Foods	Examples
Spicy foods	Includes Mexican, Italian, and curry; other spices, such as cinnamon and ginger
Alcohol	All except a moderate amount of wine
Coffee	Some folks can tolerate small amounts; decaffeinated coffee must be tested carefully
Chocolate	In any form of candy; hot chocolate for many people
Raw vegetables	Corn, cabbage, beets, popcorn
Stringy meats	Stew meats, pot roast, Swiss steak, etc.
Nuts and seeds	Peanuts, almonds, sesame seeds; even seeds in rye bread cause trouble. (Many people identify nuts as a serious problem. It could be that the pieces of nuts cause irritation. You might test peanuts versus smooth peanut butter.)

Foods	Examples
Fatty meats	Includes steak, beef, pork
Diet beverages	This includes carbonated and noncarbonated
Raw unpeeled fruits	Unpeeled apples, peaches, pears, and grapes
Sugar	Foods that contain a lot of sugar, such as cakes, icing, or soft drinks
Additives	Monosodium glutamate (MSG), possibly saccharine for some
Processed meats	Sausage, cold cuts such as bologna, salami, etc., and frankfurters
Dairy products	This is variable; whole milk, ice cream, and some cheese; a small amount of low-fat milk is all right, especially on cereal
Desserts	Ice cream, cream pie, cheesecake, chocolate
Shellfish	Many people can't eat shellfish, such as clams, oysters, and mussels; they can't eat crustaceans, such as shrimp, lobster, and crabs

TABLE 2.2
Food Preparation Methods that Cause Flare-ups

Pickling: Pickled vegetables, such as sauerkraut, pickles, relishes.

Gravy: Meats that are well-tolerated, such as chicken and turkey, can cause flare-ups when gravy is added.

Uncooked Vegetables: If some vegetables are cooked well, they're all right.

Frying: Foods that are well-tolerated, such as fish, will cause flare-ups if they're deep-fat fried or even pan-fried in oil.

Charcoal Broiling: Beef or other meats that are barbecued are fine as long as they're not seared or charred.

CHAPTER THREE

Creating a Food
and Lifestyle Diary

There are several ways to find out what causes your flare-ups. The simplest and most direct way is to keep a food and lifestyle diary. It doesn't cost much, takes very little time, can be done without supervision, and pays big dividends. And people who use a food lifestyle diary usually learn as much about themselves as what causes flare-ups.

Self-Health Management

Your doctor is the most expensive contractor you hire. The doctor's value to you depends on the quality of information you provide. The more you know about your body, about how it works and responds, the more effective he'll be when you need him. I call this concept "self-health management."

This is the way it works. Let's say that about two or three days after you eat tangerines you get small, cankerlike sores inside your mouth; a few days later, cramps, then a full blown flare-up. It wouldn't take long to associate the mouth sores with the flare-up, but the tangerines could take much longer. In fact, your doctor is likely to detect the mouth sores, but not that you've eaten the tangerine.

If you'd like to refine your instinct, you might try canned tangerines; they're likely to have the membranes removed. These membranes are rich in bioflavinoids, a group of materials that could conceivably cause the flare-up. Or you might wonder, will mandarin oranges do it? Better still, if the mouth sores precede the flare-ups by a few days, is it possible to avoid the flare-up? You might want to experiment with some supplemental fiber, for example Metamucil taken as a supplement.

The concept of self-health management doesn't stop with food. Suppose that between the mouth sores and the flare-up there is some emotional upset, or that the flare-up is not caused by tangerines alone, but also some stress, or as many people say, "fatigue." The only way you'll ever be able to know for sure is to keep a good record and to discuss it with health professionals. It's also useful to discuss the problem with a self-health group. You might get some excellent ideas from your peers. After all, they live with the illness every day as you do and no one else can relate in quite the same way.

Jean has Crohn's disease. She was having flare-ups in the form of cramps followed by diarrhea. The doctor prescribed some medication. It worked, but the price was drowsiness and dry mouth—a real drag on her life. I noticed she drank a large glass of milk with just about every meal, and I asked her why. "Habit," she said. I suggested an alternative for the next ten days. "Eat oatmeal every morning with fruit yogurt blended in, a sort of muesli, and don't drink any milk at all."

She stopped the medication, the cramps stopped, the diarrhea slowed down, and all her meals were more enjoyable. She didn't feel drowsy and didn't complain of dry mouth. Of course, I had guessed at the milk, and knew that oatmeal is a good source of soluble fiber; it helps to slow the action of the small intestine. She could have identified both the problem and the solution ten years ago. I asked her a simple question: "Did you ever tell the doctor about all the milk you drink?"

"No," she said.

I ask, "Why?"

The answer: "He didn't ask."

Think of how much more helpful her doctor would have been and how much better she would have felt if she'd kept a food diary. If she had practiced self-health management she could have provided the doctor with complete information. Her doctor could have suggested alternative approaches and they'd both have been better off. They could have learned from the experience.

As a sequel, Jean started using the fiber supplement Metamucil once daily with her doctor's consent. She now has fairly normally bowel movements and only occasional diarrhea. She uses Lactaid milk.

Sensitivity Versus Allergy

In recent decades scientists recognized that some people have sensitivities to foods. These are not allergies; people don't break out with a severe rash or get swollen eyes. Rather, these sensitivities show up in very subtle ways—for example, a headache, congestion or a little nausea.

Another characteristic of sensitivities is the threshold. In contrast to an allergy, a sensitivity sometimes doesn't emerge until you eat a certain amount of the food. It's as though your body has to get enough to realize it's got something it doesn't like. For example, you might be able to eat one egg, but not two. Or you might be able to eat an egg today and another one tomorrow, without ill-effect, but if you eat an egg on the third day, watch out. By contrast, if you're allergic to eggs and you eat one, you'll know it. You might break out into a rash or get sick; or you'll react if it's an ingredient in something you ate. In other words, a sensitivity is not an allergy.

That's why I urge anyone with IBD to keep a food diary. It helps you identify food sensitivities and puts you in control. You're the only one who can do it, because you're the only one who knows how you feel.

Keeping a Food Diary

A food diary is a simple thing. You keep track of what you eat or drink, where, when, how much, why, and how you felt at the time. Then at the end of the day, you critique what you ate and how you feel. List the number, types, and consistency of bowel movements, and also write down any other important observations that relate to how you feel or how you look.

Record how you feel emotionally. Is there something that caused you stress, anger, or fear, or simply upset you? Write it down. Sometimes patterns emerge that will allow you to avoid sources of stress. We'll talk more about this in Chapter Twenty-two.

Keep a record of your body and how you're feeling, because IBD flare-ups often start in subtle ways—with canker sores, for example, or red nodules, or bloodshot eyes. If you can relate to the signs of an oncoming flare-up to food, or an emotional experience, you'll be able to manage your illness more effectively. Your doctor will be delighted if you could say as Barbara did, "Every time I eat tangerines I get canker sores and if I don't stop, flare-up follows." Your doctor would say not to eat tangerines, but would want you to keep the diary and find other flare points. I would be surprised if it's only tangerines.

You might ask: "Why does Dr. Scala suggest I keep track of where I eat?" The answer is simple. Some food establishments use methods of preparation or ingredients in their food that aren't obvious to the customer. For example, they might use meat tenderizers, a spray to keep their lettuce looking fresh on the salad bar, or a flavor enhancer in sauces. If you got a flare-up within a few hours, a day or so, or even a week after you ate at a certain restaurant, you'd be in control, able to try another meal selection, have it prepared especially for you, or find another restaurant. You'd be in control and wouldn't be feeling depressed about an unknown cause. Your doctor would be pleased as well.

Details of the Diary

There's no established way to keep a food diary. After working with several groups of people who suffer from arthritis, asthma, and other illnesses, I can tell you what works best from experience. It's easy.

Start by purchasing a spiral notebook, one that is at least 9½ inches by 6 inches. I prefer the standard 8½ inches by 11, but the smaller one fits in pocketbooks, so it's more convenient. People who carry a briefcase could use the larger size. Whatever works is okay.

Date each page and start by noting how you feel when you get up. Morning is important because during the day, in the midst of our daily activities, we often suppress feelings of discomfort. More, when we're active, our brain produces chemicals called endorphins. Endorphins, also called "natural opiates," have a mood-lifting effect; they make us feel good. We're likely not to recognize mild discomfort when our brain is producing endorphins. In the morning, the previous day's endorphins are gone, so we start to feel our discomforts again.

Write down what you eat during the day. Be as specific as possible. If you started the day with a bowl of cereal, was it oatmeal, corn bran, or some other cereal? Did you use whole milk, skim, 2 percent, or Lactaid? How much? Did you add sugar? Be as specific as possible about food. Don't just list potatoes, for example; write down if they were white, red, or sweet, how they were prepared, and if the skin was removed.

It's essential that you record everything: meals, snacks, and beverages. There's no way to be certain ahead of time what will cause or aggravate a flare-up. In addition, a flare-up can be a reaction to a combination of foods, or the interaction between medication and a food. You're looking for anything that can cause trouble. Once you've found it, you're in control! And there's always an alternative.

Serving size or the amount eaten is next in importance after the food itself. Experience will help you estimate. Some things are easy, such as an apple, pear, banana, potato, or a cup or two of green beans. But how much cereal did you eat? You simply poured it from the box to the bowl; then, how much milk? It's easy to simply measure these things once in a while to get a feeling for what a cup of cereal looks like. It's the same with spaghetti, rice, and other commonly used foods. We seldom measure out our food, but it's worthwhile to get a good idea of how much you're actually eating. You only need to do it a few times.

If you're using food supplements, a fiber supplement, or a supplemental food, it's important to note what brand and how much. Fiber supplements should be chosen with appropriate bowel movements in mind. If you've chosen it correctly, and are using enough, the frequency and consistency of your bowel movements will be your grade. Yes, stool frequency, size, color, and even odor are important; even time after eating is a factor.

Write down where you eat, too—for example at a friend's house or a restaurant. Location is an important factor with food.

That gets you to the end of the day. Now for the critique. First note how you felt. Then identify any unusual physiological events, either positive or negative. For example, if you had seven watery stools, it's important. But if you had only one with good consistency, that's even more important, because it means you're doing something right. A major change will help you identify a problem food. Next, evaluate the emotional events of the day. If things were average, that's okay. But if there was some unusual stress or emotional upheaval, identify it, analyze it, and remember it, because if you wake up tomorrow or the next day feeling sick, it could be the cause. Along with food, the emotional upset could be part of the cause of your flare-up.

Finally, grade your food selection. How did you do nutritionally? Did you get everything you needed from your food? Did your supplements provide general nutrition and make up for specific shortfalls, such as calcium? If you took fiber supplements, were they enough? You're trying to get maximum benefit from food and should strive to get it right.

Write down every change in your body. Did you get a canker sore? Notice a rash? Sometimes the preliminary indicators of an intestinal upheaval are nonintestinal flare-ups—canker sores, red nodules on the arms or legs, sores anywhere on the body. They're important for two reasons. First, when you learn to identify them, they serve as your early warning. They provide the first clue to any food initiators of your flare-up. Second, once you learn what caused them, you have learned what triggers an intestinal flare-up. You can, therefore, eliminate a food or source of stress that causes an intestinal reaction. It's self-health management.

When a Food Causes a Reaction

Let's say you've used a food diary and some food you've eaten causes a serious reaction. Should you eliminate it? No, not until you've tested it a couple of times under different circumstances. Suppose you eat brussels sprouts with foods you know are safe, and you end up with a long bout of diarrhea or a case of abdominal cramps. Let things return to normal, then try again using a small amount with a food you know is bland—like mashed potatoes. If you get a reaction, it's probably the brussels sprouts, but I recommend one more try with a similar small amount and another safe food. If you get a reaction, then you can put it on your list of foods to avoid.

It's probably worthwhile to return to these foods in a year

or two to see if they're still a problem. Food sensitivities have a way of slowly changing, so you must keep testing.

Food Diary Versus Elimination Diet

Some doctors use what they call an "elimination diet." This is a program in which certain foods are added and some eliminated. It's excellent for identifying food groups and even specific foods that cause trouble. For example, suppose you have chronic diarrhea. You eliminate all wheat-containing foods and the diarrhea clears up. You could be sensitive to wheat; in fact, you might even be unable to tolerate a wheat protein called gluten. But even an elimination diet won't replace a food/lifestyle diary.

An elimination diet should be done under your doctor's supervision. There are several critical variations, such as eliminating one group before another. So, although this may sound like an easy diet procedure, it is very sophisticated and requires professional supervision.

Even if your doctor prescribes an elimination diet, maintain the diary. It'll make the entire process more effective. You'll be able to spot things that the elimination diet is likely to miss. For example, do canker sores precede an intestinal flare-up? If they do, you'll know it much sooner with the diary than the diet. So use both.

Sensitivity Subtleties

As I've noted, food sensitivities aren't the same as allergies. They aren't as obvious. For example, suppose you eat some zucchini bread you've been given and notice a canker sore two days later. Worse yet, suppose one piece doesn't trigger the sore and you have to eat it on three consecutive days in order to get a reaction. It will be hard enough to sort it out with the diary, let alone without one. Once you've traced it to the bread, you've got to find out if it's the zucchini or something else in the bread.

When people were testing arthritis flare-ups for a previous book, two women made the scope of reactions very clear. Let me summarize their stories:

BETTY: "I can eat an egg one day, an egg the second day, but if I eat an egg the third day, I can't get out of bed on the fourth day."

Now, for Betty to learn that about herself required perseverance. She had to keep a food diary. Norma's story is a little different; she had simply stopped eating all organ meats as the program instructed.

NORMA: "My daughter made the honor society and I attended the parents' dinner reception. They had chicken liver hors d'oeuvres; without thinking I ate mine completely. My knees were so bad the next day I couldn't walk. I forgot how far I had come."

Norma had forgotten how sensitive she is to meats. New habits had taken over. She had taken her newfound health for granted; the dinner reception flare-up snapped her back to reality.

I don't think ten experts would agree on how to describe these women's different reactions to food. Some would say: "It's in their head!" That's nonsense; legs swollen to the point of immobility isn't in the head. Some would say: "Allergy." I might agree for Norma, but not Betty. If they are, they're as different as night and day. Some would say, "Food sensitivity!" I'd certainly agree for Betty, but would have doubts for Norma. It's a complex problem, and I'm not sure it's of much value to give them a label.

Only two points are clear. Betty can eat eggs if she's careful and Norma can't eat chicken livers. Neither one should experiment with their sensitivity any further.

CHAPTER FOUR

Symptoms of Lactose Intolerance

Do you know someone who says: "Milk makes me sick"? We all do. About 80 percent of the world's population can't drink milk after early childhood or late teens. When they do, they get abdominal pain, feel bloated, sometimes become nauseated, and are subject to diarrhea. The pain usually starts as bloating, followed by cramps, waves of nausea, and then diarrhea. These symptoms, when traced back to milk, are the result of *lactose intolerance*.

Lactose is milk sugar, a disaccharide, made from one unit each of glucose and galactose. Galactose is found only in milk sugar; it's the major carbohydrate in all mammalian milk, including human milk. You could logically ask, "How can people get sick from something in their mother's milk?"

Who Is Lactose Intolerant?

With few exceptions, everyone is born with the ability to digest lactose. As infants our small intestine has an enzyme,

55

lactase, that breaks lactose into glucose and galactose. Each sugar is then absorbed from the small intestine into the blood and broken down to provide energy and a source of carbon from which to make other materials. But because of their genetic makeup, some people lose the ability to make the enzyme lactase shortly after being weaned from their mothers. Others, mostly Caucasians, lose the ability as adults, especially if they stop drinking milk.

Most blacks, Orientals, and many Mediterranean people, such as Greeks, Jews, and Italians, start to lose the enzyme lactase at about age 4; by the time they're teenagers the enzyme's gone. Caucasians from northern Europe have often lost the enzyme by age 35 or 40 because they've stopped drinking milk; if they keep drinking milk, the enzyme will stay with them.

People with IBD are often lactose intolerant. People with another illness, often called the diarrhea disease in Europe and Scandinavia, are often lactose intolerant. These people can't drink milk. If they're not aware of this, they have chronic diarrhea.

Lois's Story

I've traveled approximately 12,000 miles on speaking tours with Lois. Lois is an attractive young woman who has Crohn's disease. I noticed that she usually included a glass of milk at every meal. After drinking her milk and before the meal was finished, Lois usually took at least one trip to the lavatory.

I suggested that Lois not drink the milk for at least one week. The trips to the lavatory during meals stopped. I asked her if she noticed the difference. In her own words: "Yes. I never realized that milk was doing that." "Did you ever get cramps, or feel nauseated?" I asked. "No," was the reply.

Lois offers another example of why anyone with a chronic illness, especially an intestinal disorder, should keep an accurate food diary. If Lois had taken an aggressive attitude toward her own health, she would have related milk to diarrhea and either searched for an alternative or planned a diet without milk. Instead, she subconsciously adapted to the diarrhea that followed the milk.

Using Lactose Intolerance to Advantage

While working on drug-abuse programs I've talked with many users. A common problem among them is constipation, which develops from the drugs and is probably aggravated by a poor diet consisting of low-fiber foods. I asked one young man how he dealt with this problem. His reply was startling. "Simple, my man," he replied. "I just drink about a pint or two of milk; then boom!" He smiled. "No more constipation." That's what I call using lactose intolerance to advantage.

In contrast, at a recent lecture on third-world malnutrition, the lecturer showed a picture of a clergyman giving black children in Ethiopia one-pint containers of milk. The lecturer, a physician, then pointed out that the milk was enough to give each child cramps and diarrhea. How easy our good intention can go awry! (In defense of the clergyman, the food program was in place before lactose intolerance was understood.)

An Inborn Error or a Survival Mechanism?

Many scientists call lactose intolerance an inborn error of metabolism. That's a myopic view based on the assumption we're supposed to drink milk for life. In parts of the world where lactose intolerance occurs naturally, it is usually better not to drink milk. In hot climates, milk carried many germs, the most deadly of which was tuberculosis before pasteurization was discovered. Therefore, the inability to digest lactose helped these children survive. Only the temperate and cool parts of the world are suited to consumption of cow's milk, because it can easily be kept cool. Consequently, when someone tells you that lactose intolerance is an inborn error of metabolism, please inform that person they're wrong!

What About Cheese and Yogurt?

Fermented dairy products solved two problems very nicely. Most of the lactose is fermented and other sugars are produced; the protein and calcium of milk is still there. Everyone wins. You can eat yogurt and cheese with no side effects. Cheese is a little high in calories and fat, so it should be used in moderation, but yogurt is an excellent alternative. It can even replace milk on cereal.

Lactase: Technology to the Rescue

Why not simply add the enzyme lactase to milk and break down the lactose to glucose and galactose? That's exactly what some people do. If you're lactose intolerant, you have three alternatives. They are sold under the brand name of Lactaid.

Lactaid brand milk is treated at the dairy with the enzyme lactase, which breaks the lactose down into glucose and galactose. It is sold in most supermarkets. More than 70 percent of the lactose has been eliminated; the remaining 30 percent should not be a problem. Eight ounces of milk contain about 6 grams of lactose. If 70 percent is broken into glucose and galactose, only 1.8 grams of lactose remain—not enough to cause a reaction in most lactose-intolerant people. If the remaining 30 percent of lactose is a problem, however, it can be totally eliminated by adding Lactaid Lactase Drops.

Lactaid Drops is a liquid preparation of the enzyme lactase. When added to milk, these drops eliminate more than 99 percent of the lactose. So, if you're lactose intolerant and use Lactaid Drops according to the directions, you can drink milk! There will be no symptoms of lactose intolerance and you'll get all the nutrition that milk can provide.

There's still one more option. *Lactaid Caplets* is a preparation of the enzyme lactase and is designed to work in the human stomach and small intestine. You simply take from one half to three caplets at the beginning of a meal, depending on the amount of milk you intend to drink. That's all there is to solving lactose intolerance. No reaction.

In Chapters Five and Fourteen I make the point that there's an advantage to eating a cereal rich in soluble fiber daily. Oatmeal is an excellent choice, but like all cereals, it is generally eaten with milk, although it can be enjoyed with yogurt, apricot nectar, or some other juice. To get the benefits of oatmeal and the convenience of milk, Lactaid is the answer. Whenever I speak about the use of lactase, people ask me, "How do I get it?" Information can be found at the end of the chapter.

Sugar Alcohol Intolerance

In Chapter Thirteen we discuss the sugar alcohols, including xylitol, sorbitol, and maltitol. These sweet alcohols occur naturally in most fruit, are easily metabolized by our body, and are found in small quantities naturally. However, in many people they cause discomfort when taken in larger amounts.

Sugar alcohols, especially sorbitol and maltitol, are used in some confection products and liquid-vitamin preparations.

There's no alternative enzyme preparation similar to Lactaid for their use. Therefore, read the ingredient list. If sorbitol, maltitol, or xylitol appears on the ingredient list, use the product cautiously. Don't tempt illness.

Other Sugar Intolerance

When Europeans explored the northern parts of Canada and Alaska, they came upon the Eskimos, people who live above the arctic circle. In those days Eskimos ate a diet consisting of many foods, mostly from animals and fish. None of their foods had more than trace quantities of sucrose, common table sugar. They were sucrose-intolerant because they had simply no use for the enzyme sucrase, which digests sucrose.

Eskimos reacted to sugar-containing foods and beverages in much the same way lactose-intolerant people react nowadays to milk. They slowly adapted, however, and their bodies now produce sufficient quantities of the enzyme sucrase. This enzyme allows them to digest all the sugar they can eat. This ability for Eskimos to produce sucrase gives more insight into the absence of the enzyzme lactase in other populations.

Human beings developed largely as vegetarians with an ability to detect and eat sweet natural foods. Therefore, our body can metabolize sucrose when it's available in reasonable amounts. We call the enzyme sucrase an adaptable or inducible enzyme; if we need it, our bodies adapt and make it.

The enzyme lactase disappears after age 4 in many children. We can safely assume that they don't require its presence to grow. Indeed, the inability to produce it, after age 4, in the presence of cow's milk indicates strongly that fluid cow's milk is not required for survival. There are safer, alternative ways to get the protein, calcium, vitamins, and other minerals that milk supplies.

Summary

Many adults, especially those with intestinal disorders, are lactose intolerant. This means that milk makes them sick or at least causes diarrhea. Intolerance results from the inability to metabolize the milk sugar lactose. These people lack the enzyme lactase. This problem is conveniently solved by the use of lactase enzyme preparations, Lactaid brand milk, or a combination of both. Dairy products, such as yogurt and cheese, can be eaten by lactose-intolerant people, making possible the nourishment and enjoyment of milk.

Lactaid brand milk is sold in supermarkets, and enzymes are sold in drugstores. For more information, call or write:

Lactaid Inc.
P.O. Box 111
Pleasantville, NJ 08232
Toll Free Phone: 1-800-257-8650

CHAPTER FIVE

Fiber and IBD

My primer on fiber (Chapter Fourteen) provides a good foundation, but individuals with IBD should pay close attention to how they introduce fiber into their diet, because their system handles it differently than those of normal people. In general, people with IBD tend to avoid fiber, especially cereals. But fibrous foods are very beneficial if they are properly dealt with. Careful preparation can control the problem, which is most likely the "fiber matrix."

Matrix Problems

The fiber matrix, consisting of all six types of fiber, spells trouble for folks with IBD. In many fruits, vegetables, and legumes, the matrix simply needs to be removed. That's why apples and pears should be peeled. In other foods it must be broken down; that's why some vegetables, like asparagus, should be cooked until they're somewhat mushy, and why beans require cooking to the pasty consistency.

Softening the Matrix

Insoluble fiber must be softened for people with IBD. This means that vegetables should be cooked until their consistency is very tender. Although many people like vegetables such as broccoli crisp and crunchy, quick cooking isn't good for most people with IBD. For them, it's important to boil the broccoli until the stems are soft; this can be done by steaming, but it takes much longer. This applies to all vegetables that most people like to eat crunchy, including asparagus, carrots, zucchini, squash, and other popular vegetables. Some vegetables, such as peppers, which are seldom cooked, can be eaten only with great caution.

By cooking vegetables, especially stemmed vegetables like asparagus and broccoli, until soft, you aren't breaking down the actual strands of cellulose fibers; you're breaking down the matrix. After reading more than 100 food questionnaires, I'm convinced the fiber matrix irritates an inflamed bowel and quite possibly accounts for the observation that fresh vegetables cause flare-ups.

Canned Vegetables

The canning process includes placing the vegetables in a water bath in which the temperature is elevated almost to boiling. Canners call this process "retorting"; a homemaker would call it pressure cooking. It breaks down the fiber matrix. Although this is good for people with IBD, the excess salt used in canning is a concern. The K factor—potassium content—of canned vegetables is very poor (see Chapter Twenty-one). Therefore, when you eat canned vegetables it's important to compensate for the heavy salt load with some other high K-factor foods.

Pressure Cooking

Fresh vegetables can be cooked under pressure in a home pressure cooker. This process breaks the fiber matrix in the same way as canning. Pressure cooking has many advantages: it doesn't require the salt that's used in canned vegetables to prevent bacterial growth; you can save the liquid for soup or other uses, and maintain good nutritional value.

Peel Fruit

If there's an insurmountable fiber matrix in the plant kingdom, it's the skin of apples, pears, peaches, kiwifruit, berries, tomatoes, grapes, plums, and any other fruit that you can think of with skin. If in doubt, peel the fruit; better still, if there's anything on the fruit that resembles a peel, remove it! You can't go wrong with this as a guide.

Ripe Fruit

Ripe bananas seem acceptable for most people with IBD, but every so often someone says, "I get a flare-up for diarrhea from a slightly green banana." A greenish banana is ripe, but the fiber matrix is intact. Let the banana ripen to yellow with brown spots before eating it; it will provide you with excellent soluble fiber. This concept can be applied to many other fruits, especially avocados, pears, plums, peaches, apricots, melons, and other fruit that is shipped to the store when it's firm, even unripe. This practice is good for the store, because firm fruit lasts longer on the shelf; however, it's not good for the person with IBD. Be sure to ripen the fruit at home before eating it; this may take days or even a week.

An excellent way to tell that a pear is fully ripe is when it can be eaten with a spoon. Slice it in half, scoop out the seeds and core, and then enjoy it.

Canned Fruit

Although I'm generally not an advocate of processed foods, I think canned fruit is an excellent compromise for folks with IBD. Canned fruit has been peeled, cooked by retorting, and its fiber matrix has been broken. Fruit canned in natural juice is available, so there's no concern with sugar syrup, which has been the major argument against canned fruit. Canned fruit is peeled before canning, including grapes and even tomatoes. Canned citrus fruit has the "section" matrix removed, which makes the fruit very convenient and safe to eat.

Cereals

Cooked oatmeal is an ideal cereal, because oats are primarily a soluble fiber cereal. If oatmeal is started in cold water, cooked slowly, and allowed to become creamy, it is almost therapeutic. That's correct; some people identified it as a cereal that slows down diarrhea and calms a flare-up. Very few people have difficulty with oatmeal, but if even one person complains, it's worth saying "be careful." Better safe than sorry. Similar comments have been applied to cooked brown rice and Cream of Wheat. These cereals have one similarity: they are good sources of soluble fiber and cooking breaks down the fiber matrix.

In contrast to cold cereals, high-fiber cereals, such as All-Bran, All-Bran with Added Fiber, and similar high wheat-bran cereals provide a large amount of hard, insoluble wheat fiber with an intact fiber matrix. Some studies have shown that this fiber can actually irritate the intestinal lining. And since these cereals aren't usually cooked, the matrix isn't broken down. Alternatives are the lower fiber-flaked cereals, such as Bran Flakes, Oat Flakes, Puffed Wheat, Cheerios, and a few others. Unfortunately, these cereals are generally not sufficient in fiber content to be nutritionally worthwhile.

Fiber Supplements

Drugstores have a wide selection of fiber supplements. Most of them are made from psyllium seeds and are classified as "mucilage." They don't contain the seed matrix, are gentle, and work well. On recommendation of a physician they are often used to slow down and stop diarrhea and even quell an IBD flare-up. I've listed some of these supplements in Chapter Seven.

Consider purchasing a fiber supplement. Some are actually bulk laxatives made from the senna leaf. Senna is an intestinal stimulant and is not a good source of dietary fiber. It should be used very carefully, if not avoided altogether. Others have some fiber; read the ingredient list carefully before purchasing. If in doubt, check carefully with the pharmacist or the physician.

Plant gums are for sale in some stores. The most common is guar gum, and it's the most effective fiber for slowing diarrhea. Guar gum should be used carefully, however, because too much will actually "gum" the works. If you use too much all at once, without sufficient water, guar gum can be overly binding. It's important to consume lots of water when taking fiber of any kind, especially with the gums and mucilages. Without enough water they can actually cause a blockage. I've discussed it again in Chapter Seven. My advice is to start slowly, follow directions carefully, and drink lots of water.

CHAPTER SIX

You're in Control: Essential Do's, Don'ts, and Cautions of Eating

Food selection is your personal responsibility. An enormous variety of food is available to you. There are no restrictions other than a few "Don'ts" that I'm going to mention.

I call foods you should be able to eat the "Do's," foods you should never eat again "Don'ts," and foods you should experiment with the "Cautions." Use these foods carefully because many people have found that they can cause trouble. Benefit as much as possible from the experiences of these people.

Read Labels

An average supermarket stocks from 8,000 to 14,000 different items depending on its size. Some exceptionally large markets stock 18,000 selections! About 1,200 of those items will change each year. Some of them will be replaced by new products, but others will be changed slightly by the addition of some new ingredients. Besides a variety of products, there are also regional variations. For example, our Safeway has its own bakery where you can purchase fresh-baked bread in addition to the national brands. I've noticed that some of their bread is high in fiber and some contains very little fiber. There are other variations to serve our two large ethnic populations, Mexican and Oriental. In other areas I've visited, different ethnic groups dominate and the food choice is adjusted to meet their demands. Therefore, while I can't tell you what packaged foods to purchase, I can show you how to read labels.

Food labels provide two very important panels of information: the ingredient list and the nutrition information panel. The format of each panel is established and regulated by the Food and Drug Administration. Once you catch on, they're the same everywhere in the United States, and just about the same in Canada.

The ingredient list must contain all ingredients in descending order of content by weight. Although we're mostly concerned with the major ingredients at the top of the list, minor ones at the bottom, such as spices and artificial additives, can cause trouble. Therefore, I urge you to look at them all. It's worth the time you invest, because you'll know what goes into the food you eat and you can avoid questionable ingredients.

The nutritional panel notes the serving size, calories, amount of protein, fat, and carbohydrate in grams. Then it contains information on protein and a mandatory list of seven vitamins and minerals as they contribute to the Recommended Daily Allowance—the RDA—for adults (see Appendix). Below the nutritional panel there is information on sodium, potassium, and carbohydrate, including fiber. Once you're familiar with the nutritional panel, you'll be able to purchase one food in preference to another using nutritional value as your guide.

I will take you through one food product, Post Bran Flakes, to illustrate these points.

The ingredient list is about two-thirds of the way down on

the right-side panel. The right-side panel is on the right side of the box when you're facing it.

Ingredients: Whole wheat, wheat bran, sugar, natural flavoring, salt, and corn syrup

Next the ingredient list names the vitamins and minerals that have been added. There are no artificial colors or flavors. This ingredient list tells us that the product is good. The cereal is made mostly from wheat and wheat bran.

The nutritional label tells us even more. It tells us that a serving is 1 ounce (⅔ cup). It follows:

	One Ounce of Cereal	With ½ Cup of Skim Milk
Calories	90	130
Protein	3 g	7 g
Carbohydrate	23 g	29 g
Fat	0	1 g
Cholesterol	0	0
Sodium	240 mg	300 mg
Potassium	200 mg	400 mg

From this panel you can make a calculation. First, notice that the cereal contains no fat. With skimmed milk it contains only 1 gram of fat. Multiply 1 gram by 9 to get 9 calories from fat. That means of the total 130 calories, fewer than 10 percent of calories came from fat. You could use 2 percent milk and add only 9 more to make it less than 15 percent.

Notice the K factor of the cereal's not good; that is, it contains more sodium than potassium. But with milk, it's a little better. So far the product is okay for our purposes, but I wouldn't rate it as good.

Next on the panel is the percentages of the U.S. RDA for a long list of vitamins and minerals. Notice that the cereal is fortified with iron, making it a good source of iron at 45 percent of the U.S. RDA. Calcium comes from the milk, as the right column shows, and provides 15 percent of the RDA. That's an important reason for eating cereal in the morning.

At the bottom of this panel is carbohydrate information. It's where we see how much complex carbohydrate and fiber is provided.

Carbohydrate information:

	One Ounce of Cereal	With ½ Cup of Skim Milk
Dietary fiber	5 g.	5 g.
Complex carbohydrate	13 g.	13 g.
Sucrose & other sugars	5 g.	11 g.
Total carbohydrate	23 g.	29 g.

This cereal provides 5 grams of fiber per serving; 5 grams is a significant amount of fiber. If wheat bran doesn't give you difficulty, this cereal is a good source of fiber. The fiber matrix in bran flakes has been broken down during processing so it should be safe for most people. Multiply 13 grams of complex carbohydrate by 4 to get 52 calories, which means that 58 percent of the cereal's calories come from complex carbohydrate; that's fine. Read the right-hand column and subtract 5 grams of sucrose and other simple sugars from the total of 11 grams and you'll see that 6 grams of sugar, mostly lactose, comes from the milk. If you're lactose intolerant, use Lactaid brand milk or Lactase Drops added to your own milk to convert the lactose to glucose and galactose. Sometimes 5 grams of lactose isn't enough to trigger a response, but if in doubt, use Lactaid. Don't take chances.

Now consider the nutritional label with whole milk; it would add another 30 calories and about 4 more grams of fat. Your objective is to keep intake of fat down, so choose either skim or 2 percent low-fat milk; protein-fortified milk is better. The 2 percent milk provides more protein with about one more gram of fat. It's definitely the best choice.

Chemical Additives: Names

At the bottom of many ingredient lists are some chemical-sounding names—erythroborate, EDTA, hydroxybutylated toluene, propionic acid, monosodium glutamate, red dye no. 40, yellow dye no. 5, and others. These chemicals are used in very small quantities; however, if you're sensitive to them, the amount doesn't matter. I cannot say they're unsafe because their use is permitted by the FDA, but I avoid them and think you should as well. Vote with your pocketbook and avoid purchasing foods that contain them; eventually they'll disappear for economic reasons.

Don't Foods

Before I go further, I want to point out some foods that everyone says cause flare-ups. Everyone I know who has IBD avoids them; if they're unaware of the potential danger, I tell them. Let me share them with you. They'll appear again in the other lists, but a little repetition will make them that much more obvious to you.

Chocolate of any type
Beets
Beet juice
Cabbage
Fresh corn
Cooked corn
Blackberries
Raspberries

Do Cereals

You should strive to get one full ounce—about 30 grams—of fiber daily. The objective here is to get at least one-third of your daily fiber intake of 30 grams as soluble fiber. Actually, I believe soluble fiber should be more—about 50 percent of the total. Consequently, your choice of cereals is important. In Chapter Fourteen I list the level of fiber in a variety of cereals and other foods. Look them over and see what's available.

Choosing a Breakfast Cereal

If a cereal doesn't provide at least 3 grams of fiber per serving, it's only a vehicle for milk. Further, cereals should not contain a lot of sugars from either added sucrose or corn syrup. Therefore, your selection should emphasize natural cereals. After all that, I'm going to impose another caution: cereals that provide more than about 6 grams of fiber per serving. These high-fiber cereals usually contain added unprocessed wheat bran. Read the section on the "fiber matrix" in Chapter Fourteen. I believe it's not the actual fiber that's irritating, it's the fiber matrix. That's why the more processed bran cereals, such as bran flakes, seem to be acceptable. Why take chances? Stick with cereals that are moderate in processed fiber, with from 3 to 6 grams per serving. If you want to experiment, do so with caution. I've listed Do's and Caution cereals. I've selected these two lists because cereals without any fiber are too numerous to mention.

TABLE 6.1
Do Cereals
Cooked Cereals
(Cook Thoroughly)

Barley	Oatmeal
Buckwheat	Ralston
Cream of Wheat	Wheatena

Cold (Ready-to-Eat) Cereals

Bran Flakes	Most
Shredded Wheat	Nutri-Grain
	Wheaties

Caution Cereals

All-Bran	Corn Bran
Fruit 'N Fiber	Corn cereals
Oat Bran	
Cereals with raisins added	

I've listed Corn Bran and corn cereals as "caution" cereals. Practically everyone who corresponds with me has difficulty with corn. However, I believe their difficulty is with the kernels of corn, not processed corn. Corn kernels have the intact matrix of the kernel, but it's been removed in corn bran cereals. Corn Bran is a very good source of soluble fiber and it's worth a little experimentation. If you can eat Corn Bran, you've got a moderate source of fiber and a nourishing breakfast; generally these cereals have a very good taste, too.

Do: Vegetables

You should eat at least one vegetable and preferably two with each meal with the exception of breakfast. I also suggest you eat one green salad daily; however, if the salad ingredients are irritating, or you don't want to chance trying them, eat one more serving of vegetables. Be cautious and experiment with salad additions to be sure they don't cause a flare-up; be especially careful of tomatoes, peppers, cucumbers, and other salad ingredients with skin or seeds. We're back to being cautious of the fiber matrix again.

We have an incredible variety of vegetables available to us. There's no end to the varied tastes and colors of vegetables. Vegetables provide soluble dietary fiber. They are the best sources of potassium, many of the B vitamins, vitamin C, the carotinoids, and minerals. Vegetable fiber is mostly soluble fiber (see Chapter Fourteen), which helps to prevent diarrhea, binds excess bile acids, and is not irritating. It's helpful for IBD and should be part of your dietary strategy. But because of the fiber matrix, preparation is very important.

Preparing Vegetables

It's important to peel any vegetables, such as carrots, cucumbers, and potatoes, which have a defined skin. When eating a baked potato, or baked squash, be sure to remove the skin after baking.

Cooking vegetables thoroughly in water is as important as peeling them. Boiling in a moderate amount of fluid is the cooking method of choice. Steaming is fine, but the results should go beyond crisp to soft. I realize this is contrary to what many dieticians and nutritionists recommend, but their advice is for folks who don't have IBD. By cooking past crisp to soft, the tough fiber matrix is broken down.

Beans deserve special comment. They contain lots of soluble fiber. They're nourishing in protein, vitamins, and minerals, and if cooked thoroughly, are okay for most people with IBD. The best way I can describe their consistency when cooked correctly is "mushy." This is easily accomplished without using excessive amounts of water. The best example I can give is that when properly cooked, the beans will have the consistency of refried beans—without the frying.

Beans are special. A 1-cup serving of kidney beans, with its 225 calories, provides more than 15 grams of protein; that's over 20 percent of the RDA. About 72 percent of the calories come from complex carbohydrates and they provide more than 6 grams of dietary fiber; most of it is soluble fiber. Serve beans over rice and you've got an excellent meal that meets about 25 percent of your daily protein and fiber need.

Caution #1: Bean Salads

Salad possibilities with beans are also appealing, but not for everyone. In my opinion the tough fiber matrix cannot be sufficiently broken down in the stomach for many people. That's the first serious caution. The second caution is to be very careful with the oil selection. I suggest a high omega-3 oil, such as Puritan, walnut, or avocado oils. Alternatively, use olive oil. However, excessive oil can cause a flare-up in some people all by itself. Use the old saying: "Better safe than sorry."

Caution #2: Salad Bars

Salad bars have become as American as apple pie. There's only one problem: the fresh-looking lettuce, cherry tomatoes, broccoli, and other seemingly excellent produce may have been treated with sulfate or preserved in another way to keep it looking fresh. It's hard to tell, so ask, and be aware that you won't always get a correct answer. It's not that waiters lie; they often don't know.

Sulfated food looks fresh and tastes good, but can cause problems for many people. Folks with allergies and inflammatory disease often react to sulfated foods. I recommend extreme caution. It's one of those invisible obstacles that you never know about, but wonder what happened if it affects you. That's why I urge you to keep a food diary that includes *where* you eat. It's often the only way you can find out that you react to sulfated food.

A second caution for salad bars is all the potential for bowel irritation from peels and uncooked vegetables. I recommend real caution in eating at a salad bar.

In Table 6.2 I've listed the best "Do" vegetables, "Caution" vegetables, and a few "Don'ts." The "Don't" list is short, but according to the experiences of many people, it's very important.

TABLE 6.2
Do Vegetables

Asparagus
Avocado (also a fruit)
Beans—if canned, only with molasses
or brown sugar, or thoroughly cooked
Beans, white
Black-eyed peas
Broccoli
Butter beans
Carrots
Chard
Cow peas
Eggplant
Endive
Fennel
Garbanzo beans (chick-peas)
Green beans (Italian and snap)
Kidney beans

Lentils
Lettuce
Lima beans
Mushrooms
Parsley
Peas
Potato
Spinach
Sweet potato
Turnip
Watercress
Wax beans
Winged beans
Yambeans
Yams

Caution Vegetables

Alfalfa sprouts
Artichokes
Bamboo shoots
Brussels sprouts
Cabbage
Celery
Chickory
Chives
Collard greens
Cucumber
Fennel
Ginger root
Hominy
Jerusalem artichoke
Kale

Kohlrabi
Mung bean sprouts
Mustard greens
Mustard spinach
Okra
Peppers, bell
Pimentos
Pumpkin
Purslane
Scallions
Shallots
Snow peas
Squash
Tomato
Yautia

Don't Vegetables

Beets
Corn

Do: Lots of Fruit

You can't eat too much fruit. Fruit has three advantages and one disadvantage. Except for avocados, fruit contains no fat. It provides energy in the form of the fruit sugars fructose and glucose. The fiber in fruit modulates the way your body uses the sugar and the fiber is the right kind—soluble. The disadvantage is that most fruit requires peeling and the removal of indigestible fibrous material from fruits such as oranges.

Peel Fruit

If fruit has a peelable skin, people with IBD should remove it before eating. This need is obvious for apples, pears, and peaches; but who peels grapes? You may not be doing it now, but you should! When it comes to peeling grape skins, you have to decide whether to develop the skill of a plastic surgeon and peel them with a sharp knife, learn to squeeze the inside of the grape into your mouth and throw the skin away, or avoid grapes entirely. Only you can decide which alternative is best.

Section Citrus Fruit

Eating grapefruit, oranges, and other citrus fruit seems to require careful removal of the white nondigestible, fibrous material around the sections and between the pulp and skin. This fibrous material is irritating to sensitive intestinal tissues. We're back to the old fiber matrix once again. It's quite noticeable in grapefruit, where it separates the sections. Be very careful! The only sensible thing to do is remove it before eating. The real plus from removing this material is that the fruit tastes a lot sweeter without it; the best dessert chefs never leave the fibrous material on when serving a fruit dish with oranges. By the way, I'm blaming this fibrous material in citrus fruits on a fiber matrix, when it could actually be a natural irritant. The matrix is rich in chemicals called "bioflavonoids," which do have biological activity and have even been shown to have some therapeutic properties. Some have also been identified as mild irritants, however. There simply hasn't been enough research to decide for sure. So, my advice is simple: Why take chances? It's simply not worth the risk.

Canned Fruit

I'm generally in favor of folks with IBD eating canned fruit. It's got a lot going for it. Canned fruit has the skin removed (even from grapes), it's been cooked under pressure, and the hard fiber matrixes have been broken down. Even the fibrous matrix has been removed from citrus fruits such as mandarin oranges and some grapefruit. The only drawback with canned fruit is the extra sugar in the syrup. You can pour or strain the syrup off and eat the fruit without it. Or, decide that this is how you'll get some extra low-fat calories and eat away. Canned fruit is also available with no sugar added, canned in its own natural juices. These would be the better choice but either is fine.

Don't: Dried Fruit

Fruit, especially apricots, is usually dried with the skin intact. In addition, fruits such as bananas may be dried when somewhat green. Drying does not change the fiber matrix and creates the possibility of developing some hard tough pieces. I recommend that folks with IBD avoid them.

In addition, dried fruit is often sulfated. Sulfate is an agent used to kill microorganisms—a preservative. Sulfated materials often cause flare-ups in people with other inflammatory illnesses, such as asthma, arthritis, psoriasis, and allergies. The Food and Drug Administration has required makers of sulfated foods to state on the label that they've been sulfated. If you look carefully at the label on a bottle of wine, you'll notice that the grapes were sulfated before fermenting.

The potential trouble is worth avoiding. Better safe than sorry!

Do's and *Don'ts* Fruit

I've prepared Table 6.3 to identify fruit that always seems safe—the "Do" fruit. Certain fruits bear the "Caution" label because some people with IBD seem to have trouble with them.

Fruit Juices

Juice made from whole fruit is excellent. It contains most of the soluble fiber, none of the skin or seeds, and is naturally sweet. In Chapter Thirteen I explain how the fiber in fruit juice makes the sugar more acceptable to the body. High-pulp fruit juice is excellent. Read some fruit juice labels to get a feeling for how they're made.

TABLE 6.3
Fruits and Whole Juices
Do Fruits
(always peel first)

Apples	Mangos
Applesauce	Nectarines
Apricots	Oranges
Bananas	Papaya
Cantaloupe	Pears
Casaba melon	Peaches
Cranberries	Persimmons
Honeydew melon	Plums
Lychees	Strawberries

Caution Fruit

Acerola	Jackfruit
Blackberries	Kiwifruit
Blueberries	Lemons
Cherries	Loganberries
Currants	Loquats
Dates	Mulberries
Elderberries	Pineapple
Figs	Raspberries
Gooseberries	Tangerines (peel and
Grapefruit (section)	section)
Grapes (peel)	Watermelon

Do: Lots of Fish

Fish is one food that everyone rates high. Experts, including the surgeon general, tell us fish is good food for everyone. IBD patients can eat fish without any flare-ups. It seems you've got everything to gain and nothing to lose by including it in your diet. In addition, fish has a special benefit for IBD patients.

In Chapter Twelve I explain a possible role for the omega-3 oils in reducing the flare-ups of IBD—and fish is the best, most practical source of the omega-3 oils. With this in mind, I urge you to enjoy fish and explore the myriad ways in which it can be prepared. I've summarized the fish in Table 6.4 by their omega-3 content.

In addition to the oil content of fish, the texture provides another advantage. Some meat is not acceptable for people with IBD due to irritation from some undigestible parts. This includes what we often call grizzle, which is part of the tendon's tough membranes. You generally don't find this in fish. Indeed, cooked fish can usually be cut with a fork or even pulled apart with a spoon, which illustrates my point. But, beware of bones!

Cooking Fish

Fish can be baked, boiled, broiled, poached, dried, and even eaten raw. Just don't fry it, or bread it and fry it. IBD people I interviewed had a universal comment: "I can't eat fried fish." I don't believe the trouble comes from the oil used in frying, but from something else. When protein (fish) and carbohydrate (bread) are cooked together, a reaction between the two can produce tough undigestible material. It's probably just right for irritating the bowel.

Fish Economics

Fish is expensive in a pound-for-pound comparison to red meat. But a pound-for-pound comparison is deceptive because it doesn't account for the protein and calories in each. If you think of purchasing protein per calorie, most fish provides more than twice as much protein as meat. For example, 3 ounces of halibut provides 22 grams of protein in 119 calories; 3 ounces of lean ground beef provides 22 grams of protein in 219 calories. That means that if you're seeking nutrition from your food dollar, the fish provides about twice as much, because meat yields twice the calories for the same amount of protein and the calories from meat are the worst kind—from saturated fat. Don't let the price of fish lead you away from its excellent nutritional quality.

Frozen Fish

Modern fishing fleets have shipboard facilities to fillet, cut into steaks, and flash freeze fish. Although I personally prefer freshly caught fish to freshly frozen, the latter are fairly close in quality, and the frozen often gets the nutritional edge. Frozen fresh whole fish, fillets, or steaks are excellent. Avoid prepackaged, frozen, breaded fish.

Canned Fish

Select fish packed in brine or water if possible; otherwise, drain off the oil. Canned tuna and salmon are excellent sources of protein, the omega-3 oils, and cost less than fresh. Use mayonnaise sparingly because it's high in fat and has a poor K factor. Alternatively, low-fat mayonnaise is fine (except for its poor K-factor).

Nonfin Fish: Mollusks, Crustaceans, and Cephalopods

Mollusks (oysters, clams, etc.), crustaceans (shrimp, crabs, etc.), and cephalopods (squid, octopus, etc.) should be eaten with caution. Some respondents expressed difficulty with one or all of the fish in this grouping. They are, however, excellent sources of protein, vitamins, and minerals, and they contain some omega-3 oils. Use caution and approach them carefully. If you can eat them, do.

Once again, I have to invoke the possibility of irritation: mollusks, crustaceans, and cephalopods have many tough fibrous or shell-like materials that can irritate a sensitive bowel. Therefore, people who said they cause a flare-up could be simply describing the result of irritation rather than some type of allergy or sensitivity. I'm suspicious because most people with IBD can eat scallops (not fried, of course); if an allergy or sensitivity were involved, I would expect scallops to appear on the list of troublesome products, but it didn't.

Formed Fish: Surimi

A new type of "lobster," called "formed fish" or "surimi," is available in many supermarkets. Surimi is made by forming pieces of finfish into the shape of the meat from lobster claws and king crab claws, and then flavoring and coloring them with extracts of lobster and crab to look like the real thing. I suggest that people who normally can't eat lobster or crabs try surimi; it's quite good and can be used in many gourmet dishes.

Omega-3 Oils

Table 6.4 lists finfish as "high," "moderate," and "low" in omega-3 oil content. High means from 1.5 to 3 grams of omega-3 oils per standard 3½ ounce serving; medium means from 1 to 2 grams of omega-3 oils per serving; and low means less than 1.5 grams per serving. I urge you to eat fish with the omega-3 oil content in mind. It can't hurt; some evidence indicates it will help to improve your general health.

TABLE 6.4
Do: Fish
Finfish: High Omega-3 Oils

Anchovy	Mullet
Dogfish	Sablefish
Eel	Salmon
Herring	Trout
Mackerel	

Finfish: Moderate Omega-3 Oils

Bluefish	Smelt
Carp	Sturgeon
Catfish	Tuna
Sea trout	Whitefish

Finfish: Low Omega-3 Oils

Bass	Perch
Cod	Pike
Dolphin	Plaice
Drum	Pompano
Flounder	Shark
Grouper	Sheepshead
Hake	Sole
Halibut	Swordfish

Abalone	Octopus
Clam	Oysters
Conch	Squid
Crab	Shrimp
Lobster	Squid
Mussel	

Do: Fowl

Chicken, turkey, pheasant, guinea fowl, squab, and other birds are low in fat and excellent sources of protein. Select the breast and other light meat and avoid the dark meat and wings. The breast meat of fowl—especially chicken, turkey and domesticated pheasants—is especially free of irregularities. In contrast to much red meat from beef and pork, it is uniform, smooth, and free of membranes. Therefore, if it's baked or roasted the uniformity remains. Always avoid eating skin! The skin also remains intact but is often nondigestible. Hence it's irritating to someone with IBD. Dark meat is usually taken from active muscles (specifically legs), it's abundant with tendons and sinews that remain undigested and potentially irritating.

Waterfowl is mostly dark meat, and thus, it should be eaten with caution. The breast of ducks or geese is definitely acceptable. Apply the rule of not eating the skin; remove it before cooking, if possible.

Slicked turkey sandwiches are excellent. The ideal turkey breast purchased in the supermarket is wrapped in turkey skin. Simply remove it before or after slicing. Your food diary will tell you what breads and spreads you can use.

Cooking Poultry

Bake, broil, barbecue, or boil poultry for use in salads; avoid breading and frying. Try to remove the skin before cooking, although frequently, especially in roasting, the skin left on during cooking imparts more moisture and flavor to the meat. In that case, remove the skin after cooking.

In making chicken or turkey salad the major problem is mayonnaise. It doesn't agree with some people's digestive tracts. There are two solutions to this problem. Plain yogurt is an excellent medium for diced or shredded fowl and so is ripe avocado. Although an avocado has a fat content like mayonnaise, it's rich in unsaturated oils and contains some omega-3 oils. Yogurt is low in fat and provides more calcium than milk. Sometimes a creamy, mildly seasoned salad dressing is excellent.

Don't Take Out Fast-Food Chicken

Don't eat fast-food fried chicken, no matter which state it's from and how appealing and handsome the spokesperson for the chain appears. Fast-food chicken is a high-fat, high-sodium, excessively spiced food trap. Even if you remove the skin, breading and all, there's grease right down to the bone because it's cooked in grease under pressure. It's definitely a "no-no" food.

Don't: Processed Fowl

Turkey versions of salami, bologna, frankfurters, and other traditional beef products are available in most supermarkets. Advertising tries to create the illusion that they're better for you: the "hook" is that these are low-fat versions of their beef counterparts. It's truly an illusion, because they're almost as high in fat as the beef version and they contain artificial flavors, colors, and preservatives as well. In addition, they have excessive salt. When you calculate the calories from protein, fat, and carbohydrate from these products, then compare your results with regular turkey or chicken and all-beef or pork versions of the same thing, you're in for a surprise.

Red Meat

Meat is good food. It's rich in protein, the B vitamins, and minerals, especially iron. However, some cuts of red meat are either stringy or excessive in fat. A few rules seem to help most people.

I've labeled meats in Table 6.5 as Do's, Caution, and Don'ts. Use Chapter Twelve to find the best low-fat portions of meat. Use prime meats; they're less likely to be stringy and tough. Always be sure to trim off the fat.

Do: Low-Fat Cuts

Do seek out lean roast beef, lean ground sirloin, and lean filet steak. Flank steak, the leanest cut of meat, is a possible trap. Flank steak can be stringy (Chapter Eleven) and it requires marinades that might be overly spicy. Proceed with caution; however, it's worth preparing a mild marinade and sauces because flank steak is a good, low-fat cut of meat.

Don't: Organ Meats

Organ meats are high in fat. The brain is just about all fat. If there's any single group of foods that clearly belongs in the "Don't" category, it's the organ meats from beef, lamb, or pork.

Don't: Processed Meats

Avoid processed meats, such as bologna, salami, frankfurters, and sausages. They're excessive in saturated fat, full of nitrates and other preservatives, and salt. Most people avoid them because they cause flare-ups; they're also not good for your heart and arteries. Indeed, no adult should consume any of these products.

Cooking Meat

Broiling and roasting meat are definitely safe methods. Barbecuing appears to be all right if the meat isn't charred. Rare beef, or any blood-red meat seems to present a problem. I suspect that some of the membrane material can't be digested until it's cooked. Therefore, I recommend the meat be cooked to a pink; a chef would call it "medium." Don't fry meat; as we've seen, any fried food seems to cause flare-ups.

Portion size seems to be important, because a flare-up from food represents a food sensitivity. In my interviews many people said, "As long as I eat a small portion and chew it well, there's no problem." Therefore, the best rule is to play it safe and choose small servings.

TABLE 6.5
Do: Meat

Lean prime beef	Rabbit
Lean ham	Veal
Lamb—fat trimmed	Venison
Pork—fat removed	

Caution: Meat

Flank steak	Lamb chops—trim fat
Filet	Prime rib of beef
Ground chuck	

Don't: Meat

Organ meats	Sandwich spreads
Processed meats	from meat
Sausages	

Do: Pasta

Pasta is an excellent way of obtaining both protein and complex carbohydrate. Read the ingredient list to be sure the first ingredient is wheat or spinach. Corn pasta is not widely available and should be used with caution; it seems that IBD folks have a problem with the corn kernel, not the flour.

Sauce Is King

With pasta, sauce is king and that's where you should be careful. Most people can eat peeled, cooked tomatoes, but the spices used in a sauce can be a problem. Therefore, select mild spices, use onions, shallots, garlic, and ginger carefully and sparingly. Try avoiding a condiment such as garlic; instead use a little garlic oil made by crushing fresh garlic. Do the same with a small amount of onion or shallots in order to get the flavor and not pieces of the food. It also helps to put the sauce (after cooking) through a food processor or ricer to eliminate large pieces.

An excellent meal is pasta with a tomato sauce containing fish, poultry, or clams. Meat sauce is excellent if the meat is low in fat and is used sparingly. Tomato sauces with broccoli, zucchini, carrots, or mushrooms are also excellent. Parmesan cheese adds flavor and the added nourishment of some calcium. Bon appétit!

Caution: Dairy Products

Dairy products are a mixed blessing. They're nourishing, but they can cause problems. Many people express the problem very clearly; let me quote from Jean. "Milk causes intestinal discomfort, gas, bloating, and spasms. Lactaid makes it possible for me to use milk on cereal. I even drink a glass of Lactaid milk occasionally."

This typical response brings to the fore the most common problem with milk. Many people with IBD are lactose intolerant. If lactose intolerance is the problem, Lactaid is the answer. Read Chapter Four to gain an understanding of the problem and the solution.

Do try to use nonfat dairy products, such as cottage cheese and yogurt made from skim or nonfat milk. However, some folks have trouble with certain dairy products, such as ricotta cheese and some other varieties. To remedy this situation, keep a food diary and identify the problem; then search for a solution.

Dairy Desserts

Sherbet seems to be accepted by all IBD folks, and some can use low-fat ice cream. But many people identified ice cream as a cause of flare-ups. Therefore, ice cream should be eaten with caution. (Read Chapter Twenty-two on stress.) The flare-up could also be a response to the coldness of ice cream. Since you drink cold liquids with no problem, you might ask, "What's so different about ice cream?" Answer: the heat capacity of ice cream. Simply put, ice cream, with its extra fat and carbohydrate, can take a lot of heat away from your stomach and this could cause some stress. It's an idea that could explain the almost universal response I received identifying ice cream as a cause of flare-ups.

Pudding made with skim milk (or Lactaid milk) is an excellent dessert. Let's do some arithmetic: ½ cup of butterscotch pudding made from a mix with low-fat milk contains 4.7 grams of fat; that's 42 calories from fat out of a total of 171 calories, or only 25 percent from fat. Add some fruit, such as ripe bananas, and you've reduced the fat to less than 20 percent of calories. You can improve it even more by using skim milk. It's a nourishing dessert.

Searching will produce all kinds of dessert recipes that make use of skim milk and low-fat cheese. We make cannoli, the Italian dessert, frequently in our house. You could do the same; when you make the ricotta cheese filling, simply leave out the bits of dried fruits and chocolate chips. Remember to keep the fat calories as low as possible. By topping with fruit, you introduce more of the correct kind of carbohydrate and reduce the percentage of calories from fat. You also introduce more flavor.

Garlic, Onions, Chives, and Shallots

Use these foods with caution. They're good for you, so ideally, everyone should be able to eat them. The natural materials in these foods help to protect us from cancer, high blood pressure, and other illnesses. However, a number of people claim they cause flare-ups, so caution is the rule of the day! Be careful and test them slowly. If you can tolerate them, go ahead; you'll be healthier for the experience.

Extreme Caution: Nuts

Most people have difficulty with nuts. I suspect it's not anything in the nuts, but the fact that bits of nuts irritate the lining of the intestine. Other research on the digestibility of nuts indicates that these "bits" go through the system intact in people without IBD, so they will definitely be problematic for those with IBD.

You can certainly get along without eating nuts. If you want to do an experiment, try small amounts of peanut and cashew butter. See if you have a reaction (use your food diary). If you react to both, your problem is nuts; if neither one causes a reaction, you have evidence for the problem of chunks. If you react to one and not the other, your sensitivity is probably related to the specific nut.

CHAPTER SEVEN

Supplementation: Adding Vitamins, Minerals, and Fiber

In a book entitled *Treating IBD* (see page 370), the authors point out that a common drug for IBD, Azulfidine, interferes with absorption of folic acid, an important B vitamin (Chapter Seventeen). A deficiency can produce serious illness. In fact, people who are deficient in folic acid have an increased risk of cancer. It's common practice for a physician to prescribe a B-vitamin supplement when a deficiency of folic acid is suspected. People with IBD *should* supplement, so that a deficiency never develops. Supplements are so readily available, and so reasonable in cost compared to medication, no one should ever become deficient in any nutrient.

Supplementation of the diet by adding nutrients has probably been around as long as humanity itself. There are lots of old wives' tales to explain adding nutrients to an inadequate diet. For example, acting on "every child needs the January sun" adds vitamin D to supplement mothers' milk in the winter. Putting nails in apples or adding iron filings (from sharpening swords) to wine are ways of getting more iron. Adding a pinch of limestone to tortilla dough or making a soup stock by dissolving bones in vinegar are ways of getting more calcium. And an apple a day adds more fiber to your diet—even if you peel the apple.

Dietary supplements during pregnancy have always been popular—physicians recognize that pregnancy requires above average nutritional care and they don't want to take chances. It's called "nutritional insurance." The first supplement industry began in ancient Africa: termite droppings were collected from the sides of termite mounds. The droppings were formed into balls and sold by gatherers to other, less fortunate tribes. Pregnant women used them in their food and ate them to fortify themselves during pregnancy and produce healthier children. Termite droppings contain vitamins, but their strength is in their mineral content; they're rich in magnesium for example. Thanks to technology, we can now formulate the nutrients and press them into a pill or capsule; we needn't collect termite droppings.

Pregnancy provides an excellent example of a condition that cries out for supplementation. Why shouldn't the same attitude prevail with IBD? Certainly IBD, like any chronic illness, demands that bodies perform far beyond normal limits.

Balanced Diet

Most Americans could eat a balanced diet, but they don't. (If you examine carefully the statements of nutritionists and dieticians, they all say *can* and never use the word *do!*) Every government nutritional survey indicates that most of us fall short in several nutrients, including vitamins A, B_1, B_6, folic acid, and the minerals iron, zinc, magnesium, and calcium—compared to the RDA. Since the RDA has a safety net built into it, a person getting a little less will still be in a state of satisfactory health.

One major reason for the shortfalls is calorie consumption. Most women eat fewer than 2,000 calories daily and the intake of many falls below 1,500. Nutritionists generally agree that below 2,000 calories, the average person can't balance a diet. There's simply not enough room for error. Men have it a little easier because they eat more food and need less iron. Men, however, also consume more "empty calories." If the empty calories start to account for 10 percent of calories, a balanced diet is unlikely.

Large numbers of people fall more than 40 percent below the RDA for iron, zinc, calcium, vitamin A, and folic acid. It's not a matter of calories; it's simply poor food choice. By getting only 40 percent of the RDA they lose the safety net. Eventually a continuous shortfall of 40 percent will extract a toll on health. The term *premature aging* is often used by physicians who study and treat people who were continually deprived of good nutrition, but still get by. They don't mean premature aging in the sense of being too fat and having poor cardiovascular health. They mean that systems aren't as viable, so there's a greater tendency to wrinkles or getting prematurely gray.

IBD makes a balanced diet very unlikely. In my discussions with IBD patients I was impressed by how they learned to avoid foods that cause discomfort. But by avoiding certain foods, they increase their chances of falling short in vitamins A, B_1, B_6, folic acid, and some trace minerals, which are usually found in fresh vegetables. Since meat and shellfish are restricted by many or not eaten at all, iron, zinc, and magnesium are likely to be in short supply. Intestinal discomfort surrounding dairy products makes getting sufficient B_2, calcium, and magnesium difficult. This probable nutrient imbalance doesn't mean that people who can't tolerate dairy foods or vegetables will fall outside the RDA safety net; it means that the IBD sufferer is more vulnerable to dietary imbalance than the average American. Add to that several other issues, and the situation becomes serious. The case for supplement use builds quickly.

Malabsorption

Between watery stools, flare-ups that cause severe diarrhea, living with intestinal inflammation, or having had part of the small intestine and colon removed, there's a great likelihood of below-average absorption of many, if not all, nutrients from food. One proven way to overcome this possible shortfall is simply to add more nutrients. We do this by either eating more of the correct foods, using special supplementary foods, or using food supplements, such as vitamin and mineral supplements.

Stress

I've devoted Chapter Twenty-two to stress in IBD and in the Preface I discussed the probable role of stress in the development of IBD. The stress on your body from living with a chronic illness can't be precisely calculated, but it's there. We know stress increases the need for nutrients; after all, they're the tools that help the body do what it must to compensate for stress. No one has ever put people with a chronic illness, such as IBD, in a metabolic ward and determined their need for specific nutrients. If they ever do, I'm sure they'll be surprised. We do know that chronic illness increases nutritional need; it's prudent to believe that IBD is not different.

Medication

Some IBD patients who have written or contacted me take as many as 20 medications daily (see Chapter Two). The most basic of all medication, aspirin, increases the need for vitamin C and folic acid, so we'd better think seriously about the big-league medication used for IBD. Just consider the side effects people describe: dizziness, light-headedness, drowsiness, dry mouth, dry eyes, nausea, moon face, and lethargy, to name a few. If your doctor doesn't believe the side effects are physiologically important, ask her if she believes they account for more stress. Stress alone is reason to supplement.

Look to the Experts

Two surveys of registered dieticians showed that 50 to 60 percent of them supplemented their diet. That's 20 percent above average; about 45 percent of the general population use supplements. What do dieticians know that average folks don't? I'll bet the dieticians realize that even they don't eat a balanced diet! After all, most of them are women and eat fewer than 2,000 calories daily; they simply don't want to leave it to chance.

Another, more recent study of supplement use showed that the more educated people are, the more likely they are to use supplements. Use is also proportional to income.

Cost

Have you read that supplements are expensive? Have you also read that nutrient supplements just end up as expensive urine? Let's briefly review these two statements to set the record straight.

Sensible supplements for IBD would cost from 7 to 20 cents daily. The cost of anything is relative to the alternatives. Look at a few per-capita expenditures by Americans:

- 7.8 ounces of soda each day, about 55 cents
- approximately over 4 ounces of sugar, about 12 cents
- pet food, more than 9 cents per day

I won't go into other, more harmful consumptions, such as cigarettes, alcohol, or illicit drugs. By comparison, sensible supplements would be a bargain at twice the price. Let's examine the other statement—that taking supplements is responsible for expensive urine.

Experts have concluded that the nutrients appear in the urine, which proves that they are absorbed and enter into the bloodstream. So if you need more nutrients, they're there! In the course of a 24-hour period, the body will excrete and metabolize a percentage of its vitamins and minerals. That's why when political protestors use self-imposed starvation to get attention and drink only water, they progressively become irritable and depressed, become "night blind," are irrational and weak, and suffer many other symptoms. Finally, unless they change their strategy or are force fed, they die. The early symptoms are testament to the loss of nutrients from their bodies. So, in a relative way, the urine of the starving political prisoners or anyone deprived of food *is* frightfully expensive, filled with nutrients, even though they aren't taking any in. It's much more costly than that of a healthy person who uses supplements for nutritional insurance. But the amount of nutrients excreted in the urine is not wasted. Some of it has been used to keep our nutritional balance intact.

Supplements Are Necessary in IBD

If you've got IBD you need a sensible supplement program. Most health insurance policies will pay for it. If your insurance won't pay, though, don't despair; supplementation is not really expensive for what you get. Discuss this chapter with your doctor. At the very least, tell the doctor you want to try, for a while, to see if it doesn't help you feel better.

What Should You Take?

It's probably safe to assume that your diet supplies at least 50 percent and with a little effort, up to 75 percent of the RDA for all nutrients—excepting of course, when you've got a flare-up and can't eat. I'll go a step further and say that you probably need 125 to 150 percent of the RDA that's designed for average people. This extra 25 to 50 percent is necessary because of the illness. I believe you should supplement by 50 to 100 percent of the RDA for most nutrients regularly. I say most nutrients because some of them are easy to get from food, whereas others present real challenges. I'm not thinking about protein and fiber yet; that's for later.

A Baseline:
Multivitamin–Multimineral Supplement

Table 7.1 summarizes 50 percent of the RDA for an average adult. I realize that there's no perfectly "average" person, but it's close enough to what you require. The second column shows 100 percent of the RDA. The first column would be an ideal food supplement. The nutrients I've marked with an asterisk (*) will be discussed separately because they require special consideration for technical reasons.

No supplement currently available satisfies my criteria for the ideal. A manufacturer couldn't cram enough calcium, phosphorus, and magnesium into a single swallowable tablet to achieve that level. One product, Shaklee Vita-Lea, comes close; it meets all the criterion except for the "big three" —calcium, phosphorus, and magnesium. With respect to those minerals, it provides 30 percent, 23 percent, and 25 percent, respectively. That's an excellent record and is a beneficial supplement. I use it and so does my family.

TABLE 7.1
An Ideal Supplement for an Adult

Nutrient Vitamin	Ideal 50% RDA Supplement	100% RDA
A	2,500 I.U.[1]	5,000 I.U.
D	200 I.U.	400 I.U.
E	15 I.U.	30 I.U.
C	30 mg	60 mg
Folic acid	0.2 mg	0.4 mg
Thiamin B_1	0.75 mg	1.50 mg
Riboflavin B_2	0.86 mg	1.75 mg
Niacin	10 mg	20 mg
B_6	1 mg	2 mg
B_{12}	3 micrograms	6 micrograms
Biotin	0.15 mg	0.30 mg
Pantothenic acid	5 mg	10 mg

Nutrient Mineral		
Calcium	0.5 grams*	1.0 grams
Phosphorus	0.4 grams*	0.8 grams
Iodine	75 micrograms	150 micrograms
Iron	9 mg	18 mg
Magnesium	200 mg*	400 mg
Copper	1 mg	2 mg
Zinc	7.5 mg	15 mg
Selenium	50 micrograms[2]	100 micrograms
Manganese	[2]	

[1] I.U. stands for International Units.
[2] Selenium and manganese don't have an RDA; they have a safe and effective range.
*The value here is the midpoint of that range.

Nonideal Supplements

Other supplements, while falling far short in providing adequate calcium, phosphorus, and magnesium, provide 100 percent of the RDA or more for all the other nutrients. Indeed, some of them provide very large levels of B_6, C, and one or two other nutrients. These supplements are fine; simply follow the concept of nutrition insurance by taking one each day. It can't hurt and can only help. I like Vita-Lea because one tablet a day will put you within striking distance of the RDA for everything, including the minerals. Two per day guarantees the baseline! The alternates, which I've also listed, are fine too. Table 7.1 is self-explanatory. Consider what it says carefully.

The Big Three: Calcium, Phosphorus, and Magnesium

If you drink two glasses of milk or use it on cereal, or eat the equivalent in yogurt, you'll get enough calcium so that the supplement I described will take care of the rest. A variety of foods will get you another 25 percent of your calcium requirement. For example, an 8-ounce glass of milk provides 300 milligrams of calcium, and 8 ounces of yogurt delivers 415 milligrams. If you drink two glasses of milk and eat any natural foods, you'll get at least 70 percent of the RDA. Add at least 25 to 50 percent from a supplement and you're safe. If you drink any other milk, eat cheese, or use both milk and yogurt, you'll get more than the RDA.

Some scientists argue that women need more than 800 to 1,000 milligrams of calcium daily. Indeed, they argue for 1,200 to 1,500 daily. Some make a case for men as well. This higher requirement needn't be considered here, except to say it strengthens the case for calcium supplements. Actually, achieving those levels can't be done without them.

Magnesium is another matter. We get about 30 milligrams

of magnesium per serving of meat, milk, fish, and from some vegetables, such as beans. Our average daily magnesium intake from these various sources is about 200 milligrams to 300 milligrams; that leaves an average shortfall of from 100 to 200 milligrams. Therefore, sensible supplementation of magnesium is appropriate.

Forget about phosphorus. Unless you're a vegan vegetarian —that's someone who eats no animal products at all—you'll never fall short of phosphorus. Meat, fish, vegetables, and soft drinks are rich sources of phosphorus. In fact, there's a concern among some health scientists that we get too much phosphorus. They argue that excess phosphorus causes calcium excretion and since calcium is marginal among many Americans, there's a good chance it contributes to the excessive amount of osteoporosis among Caucasian women in our society. But for our purposes, this means we don't need to worry about getting enough phosphorus.

We do need more calcium and magnesium. I favor a supplement that contains both of these minerals. They're very important for our health. Magnesium is poorly absorbed by the normal human intestine. So how well is it absorbed in folks with IBD? Supplementation with magnesium makes a lot of sense. It's truly insurance.

Why not use a calcium supplement that also provides magnesium? They are available in drugstores, supermarkets, and health food stores. I've listed a few in Table 7.2 to help you select these all important nutrients.

One point that should be made clear is that calcium is absorbed more effectively in the presence of food, because it requires carbohydrate for absorption; magnesium is similar. The answer to this need is easy: take your calcium and magnesium supplement at mealtime. Just remember, "food supplement" means "to supplement food."

TABLE 7.2
Multivitamin–Multimineral Supplements

Supplement	Company	Comments Per Tablet
Vita-Lea	Shaklee Corporation 444 Market Street San Francisco, CA 94111	50% U.S. RDA Calcium 30% Magnesium 25%
Centrum	Lederle Div. American Cyanamid Pearl River, NY 10965	100% U.S. RDA Calcium 16% Magnesium 25%
Theragran M	E. R. Squib and Sons Princeton, NJ 08540	100% U.S. RDA Calcium 4% Magnesium 25%
Myadec	Parke Davis Div. Warner Lambert Co. Morris Plaines, NJ 07950	100% U.S. RDA Calcium 7% Magnesium 25%
Geritol Complete	Beechum Products Pittsburgh, PA 15230	100% U.S. RDA Calcium 16% Magnesium 25%

Calcium-Magnesium Supplement

Calcium-Magnesium	Shaklee Corporation 444 Market Street San Francisco, CA 94111	Calcium 12.5% Magnesium 25%

Vitamin C

Stress—physical, environmental, or emotional—increases the need for vitamin C. In addition, many medications increase the need. You will usually get your RDA of vitamin C from your food and the multivitamin supplement. However, I recommend an additional dosage ranging from 250 to 500 milligrams daily. This will meet all possible needs and is completely safe. Indeed, some people take much more than that, and many scientists recommend even more. My recommendation is conservative, but I believe it will satisfy most conditions.

There's a serious debate among scientists about our need for vitamin C. Some say we need much more than the RDA's 65 milligrams. I believe we need from 100 to 250 milligrams daily. Others argue for 500 milligrams. The debate will continue into the next century. In the meantime, make sure you get a little extra for the reasons I gave; they're not debatable.

Fiber Supplements

There is no set requirement for dietary fiber. In Chapter Fourteen, I point out that a consensus of the panel of scientists is a recommendation from 35 to 45 grams of fiber. Some research done in England suggested that the diets of people with IBD are especially low in fiber. Subsequent research in which fiber was added didn't prevent the illness, but it seemed to relieve the symptoms. It's one of those things that can do a lot of good and certainly can't hurt, so why not try it? Just be sure it's not in matrix form.

The panels recommend about three times as much hard, insoluble fiber as soft, soluble fiber for average individuals. But as we'll see in Chapter Fourteen, people with IBD don't tolerate hard fiber as well as soft. So let's change the rule slightly and lean more toward soft fiber.

Table 7.3 identifies some fiber supplements that are easily purchased. The next question is how much to use. My discussions with IBD patients lead me to conclude that, if anything, they take in less than the American average of under 15 grams of fiber daily. Therefore, I would recommend a daily supplement of at least 5 grams, consisting of a mixture of soluble and insoluble fiber or soluble fiber alone. That will increase your average by 30 percent. A 30 percent change should have a definite effect. Indeed, it should help slow down production of stools and reduce diarrhea. That will help with the absorption of all nutrients. But be careful!

TABLE 7.3
Fiber Supplements

Product	Company	Type of Fiber
Metamucil	Procter & Gamble Cincinnati, OH	Soluble fiber psyllium husk
Correctol[1]	Plough, Inc. Memphis, TN 38151	Soluble psyllium husk[1]
Fiberall	Rydell Labs Inc. Racine, WI 53403	Soluble psyllium husk
Laci Le Bean	Nutrition Products P.O. Box 4676 Fresno, CA 93744	Soluble psyllium husk
Bio Guar[2]	Bio Resource Div. of Hauser Kuhrts, Inc. Santa Barbara, CA 93103	Guar gum[2]
Daily Fiber Blend	Shaklee Corporation 444 Market Street San Francisco, CA 94111	Blend of soluble and insoluble fiber

[1]Correctol contains calcium. It isn't recommended because it also contains artificial colors and aluminum.
[2]Guar gum is a form of soluble fiber that could be excellent. However, it should be used sparingly at first. I recommend only 1 teaspoon daily, working slowly to the full recommended serving.

Caution with Fiber!

A word of caution: start slowly with fiber and work up to the desired level. The typical fiber supplement is a grainy powder and calls for a tablespoon dissolved in water. If you haven't been using a fiber supplement, start with a teaspoon and increase it to two after a few days or a week; then add one more teaspoon after another week. Work up to a full serving in three weeks. If the results are good, increase the supplement until you've achieved good stool consistency— firm stools, light brown in color, and easy to pass.

Is Fiber Always Good?

No, it's not! Sometimes IBD is so bad that the inflamed intestine becomes so small that it would be difficult to pass a knitting needle through it. While the situation might benefit from a fiber supplement, I recommend caution. Consult with your doctor. The majority of people I've spoken with don't experience severe inflammation except during a serious flare-up, when they're usually under a doctor's care. That's the time to look at supplement foods.

The time to try fiber supplements is during periods of remission, when things are normal. It might help to firm up stools, stop diarrhea, and help you to feel better—or even prevent another flare-up.

Do More Vitamin-Mineral Supplements Help?

I'm often asked, "What supplements should I take?" I answer with a basic description of the general supplement plan in this chapter, then point out that there are other nutrients that people often take. Indeed, people in the audience often tell of their experiences with other supplements. Obviously, if they tell about it, they usually have realized a benefit. I'll review the supplements that are often used:

B Complex: A supplement containing the B vitamins in a single tablet is often used. The amount ranges from 100 percent of the RDA to more than 500 percent. People who do this claim they feel better, don't feel as tired, and have more energy. Or, they feel that they can handle stress better and avoid getting depressed.

There's little information in the scientific literature to support this anecdotal claim, except the fact that the B vitamins are essential to basal metabolism and energy utilization. It's understandable that if absorption is poor and metabolism is high, extra B vitamins could help. If you use extra supplemental B vitamins, read Chapter Seventeen, so you'll know which ones to look for. Then look at the balance of the vitamins in the supplement. With the exception of folic acid, B_{12}, and biotin, they should all be approximately the same. For example, they should all be the same at 100 percent, or even 500 percent of the RDA, or some other level. Avoid products in which the levels of vitamins range from 100 to 6,000 percent, or even wider. Balance is important, especially when it's in multiples of the RDA. In nutrition, teamwork is important.

Vitamin E: A number of people said they take from 100 to 1,000 additional International Units of vitamin E daily. Most of them said they did so to help the scar tissue from an operation clear up. Hanna put it in the words of her doctor: "Hanna, the stricture is gone." The doctor then got a second, verifying opinion and said, "You're a living testimony to your supplements."

Zinc: There's been a lot of press about zinc being important to promote healing. I'm not surprised that some folks take from 100 to 300 percent of supplemental zinc daily. My only concern here is that they should make sure they get a basic supplement that contains the copper described in Table 7.1. Too much zinc can deplete copper, so it's important to get sufficient copper each day.

Other Forms of Supplements

Chewing: Liquids

Some people pointed out that their supplements go through their digestive systems without dissolving: they find them in the toilet or the appliance that collects their stools. What do you do if that happens? Don't pass them through again; read on!

A few people simply take one of the supplements identified in Table 7.2, grind it up, and mix it in food; applesauce works fine. Others take children's chewable versions of the same supplements or liquid supplements. These procedures are both good and bad news. Let me explain. I included Table 7.1 as a way of showing you what nutrients your supplement should contain and also, how much it would contain if it were ideal.

Good news: If you've got a supplement like that on Table 7.1, are grinding it up and adding it to food, you're doing very well.

Bad news: Many children's chewable supplements are seriously incomplete for adults, and all liquid supplements, except for supplemental foods (Chapter Eight), are incomplete, because it's technically impossible to get all the nutrients into one liquid product.

In the next chapter we'll discuss some supplemental foods that add vitamins, minerals, protein, and calories. These are available in liquid form and can be used to advantage. The objective of supplementation is to get a basic amount of every nutrient; not just a few. Remember, nutritional teamwork is important.

Injection

Folks who have had much of the small intestine removed require B_{12} injections; some even have the total B complex of vitamins injected. Indeed, I've corresponded with people who do it themselves at home. It's important for these folks to keep this up even if they follow my proposal and take other supplements orally. The other supplements will deliver minerals that are often missing in the injectable preparation.

Children

Children are not small adults. On a pound-for-pound basis, they need more nutrients than we do because they're still growing. Read the section in Chapter Eleven on protein for children; the recommendations there apply to everyone. How can anyone assess the nutritional need for children with IBD? They generally don't grow as well as normal children, and that's a clear indication of nutritional inadequacy.

Many experts recognize that children with IBD are especially vulnerable to poor nutrition. They recommend that children's diets be supplemented so they get 130 percent of the RDA for vitamins, minerals, protein, and calories. Obviously, the calories and protein must come from food or supplemental foods described in Chapter Eight. It also means that the children should take a vitamin-mineral supplement equal to about 100 percent of the RDA daily.

Seek a balanced supplement for children similar to the one for adults. If it's chewable, so much the better. Once children are past about age 6 or 7, they can use one adult supplement. For children, the supplemental food is even more appropriate; some, such as the shakes, are especially good-tasting. These foods not only give the children important vitamins and minerals, but provide protein as well.

CHAPTER EIGHT

Supplementation with (Medicinal) Food

Vitamin-mineral supplements in tablet form are an excellent means of adding nutrients to a limited diet. They're especially important for people who can't tolerate a wide variety of food and are likely to be lacking in nutrients but some individuals need specialized foods, foods designed either to sustain them completely or to support a diet that is short in calories, protein, and electrolytes, in addition to vitamins and minerals. These foods are medicinal.

Although these foods can be used at any time, they are usually taken under special circumstances. Most of them can completely sustain life. I'll discuss them here as supplementary foods for malabsorption, foods to give the intestine a rest, foods to add nourishment, and foods to grow on. Let's begin with a description of what they are.

What Are Supplemental Foods?

Typically, supplemental foods are available in the form of prepared drinks, drink mixes, frozen shakes, and puddings. They are designed to deliver calories, protein, vitamins, minerals, and balanced electrolytes. Calories are usually provided as carbohydrates, often using simple sugars and milk to boost the calories.

Some products use milk as a major source of protein, calories, and nutrients. This creates two challenges: lactose and fat. If a person needs calories, digestible fat is no problem. Lactose is not a problem for many people, but, some folks will have to use lactaid enzymes to overcome their lactose intolerance. Alternatively, they can mix the powdered supplement in Lactaid milk.

These products have the advantage of supplementing calories, protein, vitamins, minerals, and the electrolytes, especially the important electrolyte potassium. Some of them are designed as "low residue," meaning that they are completely digested; in fact, they are predigested and rely very little on the digestive system. But they do rely on absorption by the small intestine.

Malabsorption

When your weight declines, or you can't gain weight but want to, or if you've got chronic, watery stools like many people who have written to me, you're probably not absorbing all your nutrients effectively. This means you're especially vulnerable to malnutrition. You'd do best by eating many small meals. Supplemental foods can be very effective.

If you tolerate lactose, you have a variety of products available that make life very convenient. These range from products designed for people on the run, like Carnation Instant Breakfast, Shaklee Meal Shakes, or institutional feeding like Great Shakes. Great Shakes provides convenient frozen milk shakes that pack 230 calories, with excellent nutrition, in six ounces. This product nearly meets the criteria for an ideal food supplement as well as providing calories, protein, and electrolytes. In contrast, products like Meal Shakes and Instant Breakfast are designed to be mixed with milk. If you're lactose intolerant, that means they should only be mixed with Lactaid brand milk.

Two snacks each day from any of these products will provide about 500 calories, 40 percent of your daily protein, about 40 to 60 percent of your nutrient requirements, and are balanced with an excellent K factor for sodium and potassium. They make getting balanced nutrition enjoyable.

Foods for a Rest

During a flare-up, people often don't eat because food is often irritating, especially if it contains fiber. Some people and their physicians believe that the flare-up period is a time to rest the system. The period following the flare-up, when things quiet down, can last from weeks to months. Indeed, some people point out that during this time they live on liquids. But there are also foods that can help.

Some physicians recommend low-residue foods, whereas others advise eating Jell-O and clear broth. Jell-O and clear broth give you something for your mouth and stomach, but little nutrition. And actually, unless the broth is made especially for the purpose, it's more likely to do more harm than good because of its poor electrolyte balance. (I sometimes refer to bouillon, beef consomme, and processed chicken soup as "salt" soups!) Jell-O, in contrast, is made from protein, but it's the poorest quality protein available in the food store. On a protein scale from 0 to 100, gelatin protein registers about 28—too low to sustain life. It may do more harm than good.

Certain foods made for complete nutrition are low residue and can provide complete vitamin-mineral nutrition in 1,000 calories. Other products are available that require 2,000 calories to provide the same complete nutrition. I'm speaking about the Enteral Nutritional Products made under the Mead Johnson name by the Bristol-Meyers Corporation. I'll review a few of these products to illustrate how effectively they can be used.

Sustacal Liquid is a liquid food supplement that provides 25 percent of the RDA in 8 fluid ounces; that's a large glass. It's lactose- and fiber-free and is routinely used by athletes and pregnant women, and by preoperative and postoperative patients. In short, it's designed for people who need high-quality nutrition with no residue and without lactose.

Sustacal Powder can be mixed with milk or water. It mixes well with Lactaid milk for more nutrition, but even mixed with water it delivers more than 25 percent of the RDA for all the important nutrients (less vitamin D, B_2, and B_{12}) and has a K factor of just about three. If mixed with milk it delivers more nutrition because you get added nourishment.

Sustacal Pudding gives you some variety; 250 calories provides 15 percent of the U.S. RDA in protein, vitamins, and minerals, with a K factor of just about three. An added advantage of these foods is their fat distribution. They deliver about 21 percent of calories as fat, but with an excellent proportion of polyunsaturated, mono-unsaturated, and saturated fats. Obviously these products have been designed for nutrition.

Sustacal with Fiber is the same nutritionally complete product as regular Sustacal, with 1.4 grams of dietary fiber in one 250-calorie serving. Suppose you're recovering from a flare-up and have been using Sustacal Liquid and a limited amount of low-fiber food, or no food at all; using Sustacal with Fiber is an excellent way to start introducing some dietary fiber without the consequences that might develop by eating regular food.

Ensure Liquid is a liquid food supplement that provides 100 percent of the RDA for all nutrients in 2,000 calories in eight 8-ounce servings. It is lactose- and fiber-free. It is ideal for people who can take liquid food; it's high-quality nutrition with no residue and no lactose.

Enrich provides the same nutrient delivery and contains 3.4 grams of dietary fiber in 250 calories; that's 8 ounces. In 2,000 calories, it will deliver 100 percent of the RDA and about 13 grams of dietary fiber.

For Children with IBD: Foods to Grow On

I pointed out in the Preface that children and young people with IBD fail to thrive. Failure to thrive results from poor, total nutrition, beginning with calories and including all the nutrients. So, how do you solve the problem? Remember that pound for pound, children and adolescents need more calories. Relax the normal instinct that drives us to feed children nutritious foods, and try to make the food they do eat more nutritious. Use food supplements and the supplement foods described in this chapter.

We adults forget that children are not small adults. They're complete human beings with their own needs and requirements. Missing vitamins and minerals can be made up with food supplements. Children's supplements similar to the ideal supplement I outlined in Table 7.1 are available. But protein is different. Look at Table 8.1 and you'll see what I mean. Add to the standard nutritional requirements the same or greater stresses that are imposed on the adult, and the side effects of medication. Are you surprised that young people with IBD fail to thrive?

The supplemental foods described in this chapter should be used with children. Especially valuable are the Meal Shakes, Instant Breakfast, and Nutra Shake products. They can be used as between-meal snacks or as complete meals. Indeed, it seems appropriate to use them as mini-meals or as the beverage with food.

TABLE 8.1
Protein Requirements As People Age
Protein Required

Age	Approx. Body Wt.	Per Pounds Body Wt.	Total Amt.	Percent of Adult
6	44 lb	0.7 grams	30 grams	194%
10	66 lb	0.5 grams	34 grams	138%
30	154 lb	0.36 grams	56 grams	100%

This table shows that per pound body weight, children require more protein than adults. They also require more calories, vitamins, and minerals.

Criticare HN, Vital HN: Food That's Predigested

There's one last step before total parenteral nutrition; it's *Criticare®* or *Vital®* HN, a product that supplies predigested protein in a ready-to-use liquid. This product permits the digestive system to rest while providing complete nutrition.

"Predigested protein" means the protein has already been broken down into its amino acids, or small units of protein called peptides. In addition, these products provide elevated levels of vitamins and minerals to compensate for diminished absorption.

Criticare provides 72 grams of predigested protein in 2,000 calories, together with 100 percent of the RDA of all vitamins, minerals, and electrolytes. Only 3 percent of its calories are derived from fat that has been carefully selected from safflower oil. This means it also provides the essential oil linoleic acid. Criticare is an excellent product and is capable of sustaining life indefinitely.

Vital provides 42 grams of predigested protein in 1,500 calories and 100 percent of the RDA for vitamins and minerals. Therefore, if you're on a predigested diet of 2,000 calories, you'd get about 56 grams of predigested protein and more than 130 percent of the RDA for vitamins and minerals.

Vital is available as a dry powder that is mixed with water. This makes for convenient storage, rapid preparation—and the vanilla flavor is quite pleasant.

Criticare or Vital should be used on the recommendation of a physician and dietician, or if you feel you need nutritional support. It comes in 8-ounce bottles that make it convenient to store and to use. Whenever food is out of the question and you're told to use clear liquid, ask the doctor if you can try Criticare. You'll be getting sound nutrition that requires the minimum participation of your digestive system.

Supplemental Foods as the Complete Diet

No one wants to live exclusively on a liquid diet; most people like to eat food. However, people can live on these liquid diets and thrive. In recent years we've seen famous people lose weight on liquid diets for weeks and even months under their doctors' supervision.

Summary

Food can be supplemented with specifically designed nutrients. If enough of these foods are taken, they can sustain life indefinitely. They have the advantage of not introducing more tablets to take in addition to medication, and they're complete with protein, calories, and fat, as well as vitamins, minerals, and electrolytes. These foods and the companies that make them are listed in Table 8.2.

TABLE 8.2
Supplemental Food Products

Products Made with Milk

Product	Comments	Corporation
Great Shake	Ready to Drink Concentrated 240 cal./6-oz.	Menu Magic 1717 West 10th St. Indianapolis, IN 46222 800-732-5805 317-635-9500 (Indiana)
Meal Shakes	Add milk Can use Lactaid (flexible)	Shaklee Corporation 444 Market Street San Francisco, CA 94111
Instant Breakfast	Add milk	Carnation Corporation P.O. Box 92985 Los Angeles, CA 90009

Lactose-Free Products

Product	Comments	Corporation
Sustacal® Liquid	Convenient Ready to use	Bristol-Meyers Co. Evansville, IN 47721 800-892-9201
Sustacal® Mix	Made with milk (Lactaid) or water	(Same)
Sustacal® With Fiber	Convenient 1.4 grams fiber per 8-oz. (750 cal.)	(Same)
Ensure® Liquid	Convenient Ready to use	Ross Laboratories Columbus, Ohio 43216
Enrich® with Fiber	Convenient 3.4 grams fiber per 8 fl. oz.	(Same)

High Protein Predigested

Criticare® HN	High nitrogen Elemental diet Ready to use Predigested protein	Bristol-Meyers Co. Evansville, IN 47721 800-892-9201
Vital® HN	High nitrogen Elemental diet Mix with water Predigested protein	Ross Laboratories Columbus, OH 43216

CHAPTER NINE

Diverticulosis

Diverticulosis is an illness of the large intestine. Its name describes it well: small pouches called diverticula—visualize them as many small balloons—develop in the lining of the intestine and extend into the muscular tissue surrounding the intestine. Another way to look at the pouches is as many small hernias, where the intestinal muscles are defective and the intestinal lining acts like a tube and protrudes through the muscle wall. In this way it looks like a small bubble, or balloon, sticking through the muscular sheath that surrounds the intestine. Diverticulosis is generally a benign disease, meaning that it's not active. About 35 percent of people over age 50 have diverticulosis and don't know it precisely because it is benign. It can, however, become active.

Diverticulitis

Diverticulosis is the dormant disease; it can become an active illness called diverticulitis. This happens when one or more of the diverticula become inflamed. When this occurs, the intestine can become blocked or a fistula—a rupture of the intestinal lining—can develop. A fistula is painful, can bleed, and almost always becomes infected.

When the pouches fill with either gas or stools, they become inflamed, so the first sensation is pain. If the stool contents remain inside and become firmly impacted, they can become infected. In diverticulosis that does not yield to dietary management or to medication, only one solution remains: The part of the intestine that is afflicted with diverticula is removed. This is serious surgery and often involves a colostomy. When a great deal of pressure is generated by a combination of gas and hard stools, for example, the pouches can become filled with gas, producing pain.

From this description, a little common sense can be applied. It seems logical that once established, the way to reduce diverticulosis attacks is to make the stools soft and easy to move, rather than watery, because small stools would easily find their way into the pouches whenever pressure developed inside the intestine. This logic has been tested; increasing dietary fiber is the modern dietary approach to relieve the discomfort of diverticulosis.

What Causes Diverticulosis?

Like most chronic ailments, diverticulosis doesn't have a single cause; several factors make it more likely to develop in certain people. We call these "risk factors."

Heredity is one such factor. Diverticulosis seems to run in families, except it's not like blue eyes or blond hair; instead there is a hereditary predisposition for diverticulosis, meaning that if circumstances are right and you live long enough, you'll have a good chance of getting it. Therefore, we should look more closely at the environmental factors.

Food is a major part of our environment; it creates the environment of the large intestine. Since we decide what food we eat, we are responsible for the environment of the large intestine. As in any chronic disease early childhood is important for sufferers of diverticulosis; and since few children decide what to eat, it's not their fault if they get the disease. As adults, however, we can control the environment completely and there's no excuse not to.

Fiber is the single most important factor in the development and relief of diverticulosis. We now know that people who consume high-fiber diets from birth have very little diverticulosis. In fact, very few vegetarians get diverticulosis and among vegetarians who get it, those who eat the most fiber get it least. Those more likely to get diverticulosis eat a moderately refined diet; those who get it most are those who eat the most highly refined diets of foods that contain little fiber—white breads, cereals with no fiber, few fresh fruits, vegetables, and grains. Experts now agree that a high-fiber diet is preventive. A high-fiber diet is also therapeutic. I've illustrated both these points in Table 9.1, which shows the incidence of diverticulosis.

TABLE 9.1
Prevalence of Diverticular Disease in
Vegetarians and Nonvegetarians

	Age		Fiber Consumption
	45 to 59	Over 59	
Percent with diverticular disease			**(grams)**
Vegetarians	6	21	41
Nonvegetarians	25	43	21

Data taken from: Gear, J. S. et al. Symptomless Diverticular Disease and Intake of Dietary Fiber. *Lancet* 1:551, 1979.

Fiber Consumption
in Vegetarians and Nonvegetarians
with Diverticular Disease

	Nonvegetarians		Vegetarians	
	Diverticulosis		Diverticulosis	
	Without	With	Without	With
Total fiber	23	19	43	28
% Cereal fiber	41	33	43	40

	Symptoms of Diverticulosis	
	Cereal fiber	Noncereal fiber
Symptoms	Relieved	Not relieved
	60–76%	None

Age is also an important risk factor in the development of diverticulosis. As you get older your chances of getting it increase. This age-dependence led some experts to believe that only two factors were involved—weak muscles and time. They reasoned that the intestinal muscles in some people were simply weaker than others: with more straining at stools and, with time, the pouches simply developed at the weak places. According to this theory, the older you are, the more likely you are to get diverticulosis. The incidence of diverticulosis does increase as we get older, and it's more common in people who are frequently constipated, but it isn't a necessary part of aging. It can be prevented by a proper diet.

Another factor in diverticulosis is spasm of the large intestine. An illness called *spastic colon* often complicates diverticulosis in many people. As the name implies, the large intestine has spasms. When stools are hard and small, these spasms create pressure. The pressure causes pain and can force stools into the pouches. This starts the entire pain-inflammation cycle.

What Has Research Taught Us?:
The Burkitt-Painter Hypothesis

In 1971 Dr. Dennis Burkitt, a medical missionary from Africa, and Dr. Neil Painter, an English surgeon, published their hypothesis that diverticular disease is actually a deficiency disease of dietary fiber. It was based on their two independent approaches to the problem. Their paper was appropriately titled "Diverticular Disease of the Colon: A Deficiency Disease of Western Civilization."

Dr. Burkitt observed that in Africa, people who got diverticulosis generally lived in the cities. He analyzed their diets and found that they ate a highly refined, low-fiber diet. In contrast, people living in rural areas didn't get the disease; they ate a high-fiber diet without many refined, processed foods. Since Dr. Burkitt's original papers were published, this difference between refined and high-fiber diets has been confirmed in all parts of the world.

Dr. Neil Painter did a simple experiment. He reasoned that if a lack of fiber brought on the problem, perhaps additional fiber could relieve it. Dr. Painter explained his experiment to me one day at the Manor House Hospital: "I simply went to the local health food store and purchased several packets of unprocessed wheat bran. I told each volunteer for the study to eat a large tablespoon with each meal. They could put it on their food or make a slurry with water and drink it down. Of the original seventy-two people in the study, only seven still required surgery."

Dr. Painter selected volunteers whose diverticulosis was sufficiently advanced to require surgery. In his study they ate a normal diet with lots of fiber added from the unprocessed bran. The spoons they used were very large—about two tablespoons—so they added a lot of fiber.

Recent Research Findings

In 1928, a proposal was made that diverticulosis and irritable bowel be treated by adding fiber to the diet. But the recommendation went unnoticed and, for some reason, a low-fiber, low-residue diet became the routine method. This continued despite observations that the symptoms persisted and became worse in patients who followed the low-fiber routine. Neil Painter's experiment and Dr. Burkitt's lectures changed all that.

Research has been conducted in hospitals in many parts of the world, confirming and adding to what Dr. Painter observed in 1970. The findings can be summarized clearly and simply: Insoluble fiber, especially wheat bran, is effective in reducing the symptoms of simple diverticulosis. Most researchers have put volunteer patients on high-fiber diets with wheat bran added as a supplement or as high-fiber bran cereal; in some studies it was made into bread. Symptoms declined twice as often with the high-fiber diet as with the average low-fiber diet.

Once started, a high-fiber diet requires about three months for the patient to show significant improvement. It takes that amount of time for the bowel function to stabilize completely, and pain relief seems to require the same time period. This confirms the Burkitt-Painter hypotheses: Dietary fiber changes do not develop quickly because changes in the intestinal flora are slow.

Time often works against clinical research. A study requiring people to test both diets requires at least eight months, because a one-month adjustment is required for each test. This explains why some researchers don't get complete results; they simply don't wait long enough.

Of 100 patients reviewed after at least five years on a high-fiber diet, more than 90 percent remained symptom free. This confirms that the dietary changes are both therapeutic and preventive in the long term. In view of the hereditary nature of diverticular disease, parents who have it should start their children on a high-fiber diet, as should adults whose parents have the disease, but are themselves symptom free.

One study indirectly confirms the advantage of a high-fiber diet. In cases of patients who had surgery to remove part of the intestine and didn't follow a high-fiber diet, 60 to 86 percent of them had recurrence of symptoms, depending on the location of the surgery. In other words, surgery by itself is a short-term cure, but isn't preventive. A few studies included medication. These were done on patients with severe symptoms. A high-fiber diet with medication gave better results than medication by itself. This confirms that even in complicated diverticulosis, a high-fiber diet is appropriate.

In 1973 I published a paper entitled "Fiber, the Forgotten Nutrient." Five years later I was a speaker at the annual meeting of food technologists; a man asked to shake my hand. I was surprised and asked why. He explained that he had read my paper while in the hospital awaiting surgery for diverticulosis. He showed it to his physician and asked if he could go home and try a high-fiber diet. His surgeon said his knife was always ready and to give the diet a try. Six years later the man had avoided surgery by simply following a high-fiber diet.

What Kind and How Much Fiber?

Insoluble fiber, wheat bran in particular, works best. Based on all the studies, I recommend a diet containing at least 35 grams of dietary fiber, with two-thirds of that being insoluble fiber. That's 23 grams of insoluble fiber daily. I recommend this for an adult weighing about 155 pounds. That can be adjusted downward to at least 25 grams of fiber for a 100-pound person and upward to 45 grams of fiber for a 200-pound person. A diet with these levels of fiber is completely realistic and easy to achieve.

Since the research emphasized insoluble fiber, that means eating foods with "bran" in their name. The most convenient is wheat bran, but other bran cereals, such as corn, oat, some vegetables and grains can be used effectively on this plan. Cereal foods with insoluble fiber are listed in Table 9.2.

TABLE 9.2
Breakfast Cereals
Cereals Providing 3 to 6 Grams Per Serving

Cereal	Fiber
Quaker Oatmeal	3
Crunchy Bran	5
Wheatena	4
Kretschmer Wheat Germ	3
Golden Temple Oat Bran	4
Ralston Cereals	
Muesli	3
Bran News	3
Nabisco Cereals	
Shredded Wheat	3
Spoon Size Shredded Wheat	3
Shredded Wheat 'N Bran	4
Fruit Wheats	3
Oat Bran	5
General Mills Cereals	
Raisin Nut Bran	3
Post Cereals	
Fruit & Fibre	4
Raisin Bran	4
Bran Flakes	5
Kellogg's Cereals	
Mueslix Five Grain	4
Nutri-Grain	4
Nutrific Oatmeal	6
Müeslix Bran	6

Cereals Providing 6 to 14 Grams of Fiber Per Serving

Cereal	Fiber
Nabisco: 100% Bran	10
General Mills Fiber One	13
Millers Unprocessed Bran	14
Kellogg's Cereals	
All-Bran Original	10
All-Bran Extra Fiber	14

Cereals With Insufficient Fiber

Quaker Cereals
100% Natural
Puffed Wheat
Crunch Berries
OH's
Instant Oatmeal

Ralston Cereals
Honey Gram
Dinosaurs
Corn Checks
Rice Checks
Wheat Checks

Post Cereals
Cocoa Pebbles
Smurf Magic Berries
Super Golden Crisp
Croonchy Stars

General Mills Cereals
Crispy Wheat
Trix
Cocoa Puffs
Fruit Yummy
Lucky Charms
Cheerios
Wheaties

Kellogg's Cereals
Product 19
Just Right
Nuggets
Apple Jacks
Nut & Honey Crunch
Corn Flakes
Frosted Flakes
Rice Krispies

Nabisco Cereals
Cream of Wheat

Other Packaged Fiber Products

Food	Fiber Content
Fiber (a snack bar)	5 grams

Breads	Fiber Delivery in Two Slices
Orowheat Health Nut Bread	3
Roman Meal Oat Bran	2
Less Dark and Grainy	4
Whole-Grain Bread (Safeway)	3

Set a Realistic Goal

No matter how enthusiastic you are, don't go from the average diet of 13 to 15 grams daily to 35 grams at one time. Rather, make 35 grams your goal and develop a plan to get there in sensible stages. Suppose you're typical of most people and consume 15 grams of fiber and plan to achieve the 35-gram target. That means you will increase your dietary fiber by 20 grams. A three-week plan makes sense here; it'll be three months before you'll realize all the benefits, so three weeks to get there seems reasonable.

Going from 13 to 35 grams of dietary fiber daily in four weeks means increasing your dietary fiber by 22 grams daily in three weeks. Let me put it this way: you'll increase your dietary fiber consumption by 7 grams daily each of three weeks.

Seven Grams a Week

Week One

For the first week, eat a bowl of cereal that has "bran" but not "all bran" in its name; I've listed some of these cereals in Table 9.2. This will increase your fiber intake by about 4 grams on average. In addition, eat a piece of high-fiber fruit, such as apples, oranges, or pears. They provide 3 grams of dietary fiber. This combination will increase your fiber consumption by more than 7 grams.

Week Two

Week two requires a second piece of fruit each day. That means a second apple, pear, orange, peach, serving of raspberries, or blackberries. A second serving of vegetables and a salad each day will achieve the 7 grams that are required. In addition, include two slices of full-grain wheat bread; many deliver 3 grams of fiber in two slices. Eat it as toast, or a sandwich; the fiber's still there.

Week Three

Week three calls for a shift to a high-fiber "all bran" cereal, a third piece of fruit, and at least one more vegetable. The use of whole-grain brown rice, baked potato with the skin, carrots, and beans will achieve the objective.

You'll notice in Table 9.2 that some cereals provide 14 grams of fiber per serving! They'll get you halfway to your target all at once. You're fortunate if you can tolerate them from the beginning, because it's an excellent way to get started. Indeed, if you're willing, eating a second bowl in the evening will increase fiber to 30 percent above your target. An alternative is to use a fiber supplement either as a snack or as a way to achieve the goal.

Fiber Supplements

Fiber supplements abound. They include tablets, formulated powders, food bars, and simple unprocessed bran.

Table 9.2 is a guide to cereal selection. If you choose a 3–5-gram-fiber cereal the first week, you have a choice of about 18 cereals. Your supermarket might have a larger selection. Another 2 to 4 grams of fiber can be added by topping with some berries or sliced fruit.

Week two should include a cereal that provides 10 grams of fiber. High-fiber cereals are usually bland and call for fruit to make them more palatable. We don't use much sugar in our house, but high-fiber cereals are a distinct exception. They require dressing up. It's an excellent job for a sliced banana, or a sliced peach. Don't feel guilty about using some sugar.

High-fiber bread provides 3 grams of fiber in two slices. It's a convenient way of adding 3 grams of fiber to your plan daily. But high-fiber bread is often a local phenomenon. Finding it requires reading labels and searching for the fiber content.

Return to Your Food Diary

Now you have another of the reasons I urge you to keep a food diary. It's your only way of keeping an accurate score on your progress. You need to keep only one set of numbers. By the end of three weeks your daily fiber consumption should total 35 grams. If you have been faithful to your objective, you'll be able to plan your day as you go along. For example, you'll know when to add an extra apple, a couple of carrots, or a fiber supplement to make the day complete. The objective is to total 35 grams at the end of the day; it's part of your score. Note how you feel, the number of bowel movements, and the ease of passage. Grade yourself on these parameters and compare how you feel to how you've felt in the past.

"Flatus": Gas

A joke about fiber studies suggests that to find them you simply follow your nose. When people start a high-fiber diet they often experience gas pains. That's why I suggest you start slowly and work up to your optimum fiber level. In several fiber studies some volunteers have withdrawn because they tried to take too much fiber right away. Your body needs to adjust to fiber, just as it must adjust to any other change. As your body adjusts, the gas will slowly subside to a reasonable level.

Suppose you decided to enter a ten-mile run three months from now. You would start training slowly and work up to the ten miles. You'd train slowly because you know your legs would give out or become very sore if you started off at five miles or even less. So you train slowly and work up for the event. Increasing dietary fiber is no different. You're asking part of your body to adjust to a new regimen. Even if the new regimen is better for you, it takes time for your body to adjust.

Optimum Fiber in Diverticulosis

I've set a level of 35 grams of fiber daily for a 155-pound person because it seems right from the research. But not everyone is average. You have to find the best fiber level for yourself. That level might be 40 or 45 grams; it could be as little as 30 grams. Only you will know. There will be some bridges to cross. At first you'll feel bloated, possibly a little sluggish. You might even experience some cramps or a feeling of fullness that won't leave. These sensations will pass; that's one more reason for the food diary. It helps you find your own comfort level.

Water

Stool weight is always about 75 percent water. Since you'll increase your stool weight by 50 to 100 percent, you'd better increase your water by that much or more. I know that drinking more water on a high-fiber diet adds to the feeling of "bloat," but that feeling will pass and the rewards of extra water will show through.

If you don't drink enough water, you run the risk of becoming fiber-bound. Your objective can be defeated because the fiber gets too dry and becomes impacted. It's like having a plug of semi-moist sawdust in your colon. Drink plenty of extra fluid, preferably 32 ounces of water daily to make the fiber work better. Take the recommendations in Chapter Fifteen seriously.

PART TWO

Basic Nutrition

for IBD

In my discussions with people who have IBD, I tried to learn what they know about basic nutrition and any special nutritional requirements that accompanied their illness. I was surprised by their lack of basic knowledge about Calories, vitamins, minerals, and fiber, but impressed with how much they knew about which foods caused flare-ups. I also became aware of how little they knew about the ways in which food, supplementary food, and stress control could help them.

Why Basic Nutrition?

We all need Calories from protein, fat, and carbohydrate, especially individuals with IBD. We also need dietary fiber, a carbohydrate that yields no Calories. Sometimes people who have IBD need to avoid fiber completely. Similarly, we all need vitamins and minerals to stay healthy; those with

IBD need more of them because of such problems as diarrhea, poor absorption, loss of intestine through surgery, and emotional upset.

Teamwork in Nutrition

In the next several chapters you'll be introduced to many nutrients. For some people it will be a review, but I hope even they will gain some new insights about the basic nutrients and learn how diet can work. There's one important point however: In nutrition, teamwork is essential!

You need all the nutrients and you should get them in reasonable balance every day because they each play a unique role in our health and well-being, and they work with each other as well. It's teamwork. One nutrient doesn't work effectively if another one is missing or in short supply. If your body is loaded with one and not another, the systems won't function. I like to use the chain analogy that's easily visualized: "A chain is no stronger than its weakest link." That saying is so important in nutrition that it can't be overstated. *All* nutrients are necessary!

Our bodies are marvelous. They can take an unbelievable amount of abuse. People can survive without one or even several nutrients for days, weeks, and possibly even months; however, they'll never thrive. The worst part is that they'll never know what damage is being done to their bodies, because it's so insidious that it may never be clearly identified. Remember, experts have classified people who have been nutritionally deprived, but not to the point of serious deficiency, as physiologically older than their chronological age. This tells us that these minor shortfalls extract a price on health that isn't usually noticeable until it's too late.

Please take your nutrition seriously; you'll be healthier even if you don't notice it.

What to Look For

In the next chapters I've summarized a great deal of nutrition know-how. The information I've covered in just a few chapters often occupies entire textbooks. My objective is not to make you an expert; rather, I've tried to give you information about the nutrients you must get from food, and I've tried to make it enjoyable. Nutrition has a rich history, and some vignettes of this history help create a better understanding of the many ways that nutritional needs can be met. I hope you learn the importance of good nutrition; if you do, I will have achieved my objective.

CHAPTER TEN

Basic Calorie Nutrition

People are omnivorous. That means we eat animal and vegetable foods—fruits, vegetables, grains, meat, dairy products, fish, and other foods made from them. The historical record is interesting. One tribe in the jungles of South America lived almost exclusively on fermented grain; the mainstay of their diet was a kind of beer. Another tribe in Africa raised cattle, not for the milk, but for the blood, the mainstay of their diet. Some of these practices still persist.

People can thrive on a wide variety of diets because the essential nutrients are found in many foods. As long as these foods are consumed regularly, and with enough variety, we'll get along. When you have a chronic illness, the objective is to thrive within the confines of the foods you *can* eat. That's why we will explore the concept of an optimum diet and how to get it on a daily basis, even though your food choice is restricted by IBD.

The Optimum Diet

An average adult eats about a pound in dry weight of food each day. Look at it this way: if you took all your food each day, blended it together and removed the water, you'd be left with about 1 pound—that's 454 grams—of dry material. Several grams, about an eighth of an ounce, would be the macro minerals—calcium, phosphorus, potassium, sodium, and magnesium. One more gram would be taken up by the vitamins, and the other by the trace minerals. That leaves 450 grams, almost the entire pound, for protein, fat, carbohydrate, and fiber.

These four macronutrients are essential to health, and it's especially important to get them in the correct proportions. Nutritionists generally agree that an optimum diet—meaning one that promotes good health based on juxtaposition of protein, fat, and carbohydrate—can be obtained by everyone, no matter how unusual their food preferences are. Also required is some dietary fiber and another important nutrient, water.

This optimum diet provides 10 to 15 percent of its Calories from protein, 30 percent or fewer of its Calories from fat, and the remaining 50 to 60 percent of Calories as carbohydrate. In addition, the experts generally agree that we should get about 30 grams of fiber each day. Thirty grams is about 1 ounce; some even recommend as much as 45 grams daily. Fortunately, fiber has no Calories.

To get these nutrients into more realistic units, let's do some basic calculations.

Dietary Calorie Calculations

Protein and carbohydrate each provide 4 Calories per gram; fat provides 9 Calories per gram. So, if we work out the optimum diet for a person who needs 2,000 Calories daily, we'll come up with the following:

Protein [take 12% of Calories (c) as average]
12% of 2000 = 240 c divided by 4 cal/gram = 60 grams
Fat
30% of 2000 = 600 c divided by 9 cal/gram = 67 grams
Carbohydrate
58% of 2000 = 1160 c divided by 4 cal/gram = 290 grams

Total by weight	418 grams
Fiber	30 grams

Total with fiber	448 grams
Total for vitamins and minerals about	5 grams

Grand total	452 grams

A pound is 454 grams. Thus, the person burning 2,000 Calories daily eats about a pound of food. Since most food is about 75 percent water, the wet weight will be more than 1,800 grams; that's about 4 pounds! It seems like a lot.

Table 10.1 lists the food consumed by three different 30-year-old people: an active woman of about 120 pounds, an active person weighing about 155 pounds, and a 200 pounder, probably a man. I'll work out the Calories as shown in the table.

Table 10.1
Calorie Distribution for Three People

	120 lb	150 lb	200 lb
Calories	2,000	2,700	3,500
Protein (12% cal)	60 g	81 g	105 g
Fat (grams)	67 g	90 g	117 g
Carbohydrate	290 g	92 g	508 g
Fiber	30 g	35 g	40 g
Nutrients	5 g	5 g	5 g
Grand total weight	452 g	603 g	775 g
Approximate wet weight	1,808 g	2,412 g	3,100 g
In pounds	4 lb	5.3 lb	6.8 lb

Variation

While you're looking over Table 10.1, think about several things. Larger people eat more food because they need more Calories. If the food provides all the necessary nutrients at 1,200 Calories, it will provide them at 2,000 Calories. Two people who weigh the same aren't always the same height, and don't always have the same shape. Some seem to be full of energy and always active, whereas others seem somewhat lethargic, inactive, and pensive. Do they all need the same Calories and nutrients? No, there's a lot of variation in our requirements.

What Influences Variation?

You already know intuitively that size, shape, activity, stress, climate, and your state of health influence your nutritional needs. The optimum diet for one person wouldn't necessarily be exactly the same for another person. For example, if you're an active 120-pound woman, you might require more than the 2,000 Calories daily. In contrast, if you watch a lot of TV and you're 120 pounds, you might do just fine on 1,600 Calories. If you were to eat 2,000 calories you'd slowly put on weight. Why? Because our body stores extra Calories as fat; every extra 3,500 Calories get stored as about 1 pound of fat. So let's explore briefly where the Calories go. First start with the Calorie itself.

What Is a Calorie?

A Calorie has a precise definition. It's the amount of energy needed to raise 1 gram of water 1 degree on the centigrade scale. One gram of water is less than a teaspoon, so as you might guess, a Calorie is a small amount of energy. That's why we use units of 1,000 Calories or the kilocalorie. Kilo means one thousand. It was cumbersome saying kilocalorie all the time, so we use the word *Calorie* instead of kilocalorie. (It doesn't make any difference in our discussions, but when you look up food values and see KC or kilocalories, you'll know what it all means.) A calorie measures the energy-producing value of food when oxidized in the body.

Where Do Calories Go?

Everything we do uses Calories. Eating and digesting food uses Calories. While you're sleeping you burn about 80 Calories per hour. In contrast to sleeping if you run ten miles in an hour, you burn about 900 Calories. Let's get back to the sleeping Calories, because it makes a point. Even while we sleep our body requires energy; unlike a machine, it never stops running and constantly burns energy.

Basal Metabolism

The energy we burn to keep our system going is called energy for basal metabolism. Basal metabolism is the process that keeps our body working at all times. For example, unless you're ill, your temperature is always 98.6° F; your heart beats; kidneys continually clean wastes from your blood; your mind is working; you breathe, and so on. These processes take place as long as you're alive and account for most of the energy you use. Whether you're sleeping or climbing a mountain, the basic processes are working.

Basal metabolism varies for each of us. It's influenced by age, sex, state of health, body surface area, and stress. I'll explore each of these factors briefly so you'll see how they change, but first, how much energy does it account for?

A 120-pound woman 5 feet tall has a basal metabolic rate

(called BMR) of 1,260 Calories; if she's 5 feet 7 inches and 120 pounds, it's 1,360 Calories. Say 1,300 Calories, on average, for a 120-pound woman. Men the same size would be 1,350 and 1,450, respectively; say 1,400 Calories on average. Return to the example in Table 10.1 of the 120-pound person consuming 2,000 Calories per day. Their BMR, at 1,300 Calories, accounts for 65 percent of total daily energy expenditure! BMR is where most of our energy goes. Since most of our energy is spent on simply staying alive, let's see what increases or decreases the BMR.

From my example, it's clear that a tall thin person (5′7″) burns more energy than a short (5′0″) person of the same weight. One of the reasons for this energy expenditure is body shape; the shorter and rounder you are, the lower your BMR; conversely, the taller and thinner you are, the higher your BMR. Though only 1 Calorie per pound doesn't sound like much, it can make a big difference.

Metabolic rate declines with age by up to about 2 percent per year. For instance, a person 50 years old requires about 35 percent fewer Calories than a 30-year old person. Thus, if we keep eating at age 50 as we did at age 30, we'll be getting many more calories than we need. That's why many people gain weight as they get older even though they insist they don't eat a lot. Our perception of portion size and food needs changes slowly, because it's often part of our ethnic or family background. But our decline in BMR doesn't relate to those issues; it's strictly biology.

Metabolic rate also varies with the state of health. For example, if you are sick and running a fever, you'll require more Calories to maintain a higher body temperature. But an illness doesn't have to cause a temperature to increase the metabolic rate, for two reasons: First, the body works to eliminate the illness or overcome its effects as it does with a fever; second, your body is under stress, and stress increases the BMR. In other words, if you're sick, or if you've got a chronic illness like IBD, you'll generally use more basal metabolic Calories. As a general rule, the folks I've met who have IBD generally aren't overweight. In fact, most of them appear slightly thinner than average. Remember, most Americans are too heavy, so as a group, IBD folks could be somewhat healthier from that standpoint.

Where Do the Other Calories Go?

People generally don't burn nearly as many Calories as they think. For example, most people who are about 5 feet 4 inches in height burn about 500 Calories over the BMR in a 24-hour period. Add another 200 Calories for digesting food, and they've got their 2,000 Calories per day. Table 10.2 lists some typical physical activities that account for some of the 500 Calories average people burn.

TABLE 10.2
Calorie Costs
(150-pound person)

Activity	Calories per Hour
Resting	80
Driving	120
Housework	180
Walking 2.5 mph	210
Gardening	220
Tennis	600
Cycling 13 mph	660
Running 10 mph	900

Table 10.2 shows the Calories burned by a 150-pound person. A 120-pound person would use about 20 percent fewer and 180-pound person would burn 20 percent more for the same activities. If you're realistic, you'll see, that in a 10-hour period, you're unlikely to burn more than 500 Calories. For example, few people do housework nonstop; similarly, most joggers don't run for more than about 20 minutes.

Alcohol and Metabolism

Alcohol is between carbohyrate and fat in its Calorie content. It provides 7 Calories per gram. A 6-ounce glass of wine—that's 12 percent alcohol—provides 125 calories; 1.5 ounces of whiskey contain 100 Calories. Both provide a few Calories from the sugar they contain.

Adults can consume up to 1½ percent of their daily Calorie intake from alcohol without any adverse effects. At 2,000 Calories a day, that's about a glass of wine, one mixed drink, or a bottle of beer. Above that level, alcohol begins to have adverse effects.

The adverse effects of excess alcohol derive from its toxic nature. Since alcohol is toxic material, the body marshals all its resources to metabolize it to carbon dioxide and water. If there's an excess, it can't handle it rapidly enough and the alcohol gets to the brain, where it causes impaired function. But if you keep alcohol to less than 2 percent of Calories, you'll have no problem.

Put All These Calories Together

Let's put our Calories together to get an idea of how many we need and where they go. Once you've got this worked out, you'll be able to see how to distribute your protein, fat, carbohydrates, fiber, and all the other nutrients.

I have summarized a 24-hour Calorie distribution in Table 10.3 for three people: a 120-pound woman, a 150-pound man or woman, and a 180-pound man. This way you can see the difference in daily Calorie needs.

By studying Table 10.3 and using some calculations, you can find yourself somewhere in-between some of the examples. For example, if you weigh 135, multiply the Calories by 135, divided by 120 or 1.12; similarly, if you weigh 170 or 200. Your values will be close enough for planning. You'll see that the majority of your Calories are used to keep your body functioning properly. It's important to remember that if you want to increase your Calorie expenditures, you've got to add a special activity to your day.

TABLE 10.3
Caloric Requirements
Weight in Pounds

Weight	120	150	150	180
Height	5'4"	5'6"	5'6"	6'
	Woman	**Woman**	**Man**	**Man**
BMR	1327	1478	1588	1836
Daily activity	500	600	650	700
Assimilation	160	200	200	220
For illness 8%	100	118	127	147
Total:	2087	2396	2565	2903

How Accurate Is All This?

We live in a constantly changing environment. When it's cold more Calories are burned to keep your body temperature at 98.6°F; when it's hot, you produce sweat to cool it down. So when we conclude that someone burns 2,000 Calories a day, it's an average. That means some days it'll be 1,800; other days 2,200. Therefore, there's not much concern about 100 or 200 Calories on any single day. It's what we do on average that counts. We know if we're getting it right by whether we gain or lose weight.

Why We Gain and Lose Weight

If we burn more Calories on average than we eat as food, we lose weight. Conversely, if we consume more Calories on average than we burn, we gain weight. Notice that I said *on average.* That's because it doesn't happen in one day; it takes many days, even months or years.

Each extra pound of weight accounts for about 3,500 Calories. So if you consume, on average, an extra 35 Calories per day, you'd hardly notice it. Three or more months later you might notice an extra pound. Or you might notice that your clothes are a little tight. If it's 350 Calories extra each day, then it's only going to take ten days.

In contrast, suppose you're eating the same foods and losing weight. The same number of Calories are involved, but now it's a deficit, not an excess. The weight loss could mean that your basal metabolism has increased, which usually happens because of emotional stress or illness. If you've got IBD, the weight loss could relate to a period of diarrhea or a flare-up. The reason could be a decline in your body's ability to absorb nutrients, especially fat. I'll cover this separately as a special concern. When unknown weight loss occurs, it's important to identify the cause. If you notice that you've lost a few pounds, if your clothes are looser, think about what has happened. You've created a deficit of 3,500 calories for each pound—that's if you were carrying some extra body fat. But suppose you're a person without extra fat and you experience an unknown weight loss. The mathematics gets more confusing, but I'll explain it.

Lean Body Mass

We call muscle, including our carbohydrate reserves, lean body mass. This mass of protein and carbohydrate also holds about three times its weight in water. So losing a pound of protein drops a total of 4 pounds; three of water and one of protein. The same goes for our carbohydrate reserves. Protein and carbohydrate each require 4 Calories per gram. So once your body fat reserves are low, you can drop a pound of protein, with a deficit of only 1,800 Calories. In addition, the 1,800-Calorie deficit will cause 4 pounds to be lost, because for each pound of protein, there's about 3 pounds of water.

The reason this type of weight loss is bad is that you're losing very important body tissues and reserves that your body needs to function. We'll discuss this in later chapters. Just remember whenever unplanned weight loss occurs, discuss it with your doctor. It's important.

Special Concerns for IBD: Absorption

Three conditions in IBD make weight maintenance especially important: absorption due to intestinal inflammation, loss of Calorie nutrients due to diarrhea, and poor eating habits resulting from flare-ups. Any one of these conditions can cause unwanted weight loss; all three together can spell disaster if something isn't done.

IBD patients often have minor, if not serious, inflammation of the intestine and that causes a decrease in absorption. Indeed, some folks, who have a "pouch" or "colostomy," say that sometimes food comes out exactly as it went in. Obviously the Calorie nutrients, let alone other nutrients, haven't been absorbed.

Another challenge associated with IBD is diarrhea. Soft, watery stools are often related to excessive bile acids. Excessive bile acids cause malabsorption of fat. Lots of Americans would like that problem, but for folks with IBD, it's a serious concern because they need the Calories.

Finally, the flare-up creates a situation that causes people to stop eating. We've seen that there are some products to help you avoid this. But, if a flare-up is serious enough, your doctor may resort to Total Parenteral Nutrition—called TPN for short.

TPN is used when a person can no longer get enough calories complete with protein, fat, and carbohydrate to stay alive. It's done by completely bypassing the digestive system, using a major vein to dispense a solution that contains complete nourishment. Don't confuse it with the glucose solution you sometimes see being dripped in at the hospital; that's a temporary, short-term measure to help a person along. TPN can be used to keep a person alive and healthy for life, if necessary. However, TPN is usually used as a short-term program to let the intestine heal.

CHAPTER ELEVEN

Protein

In the nineteenth century, scientists recognized that a nitrogen-containing substance in food was essential for life and health. They called this substance *protein*, coming from the Greek word *proteios*, meaning "of prime importance." Since then we've learned that the building blocks of protein, the amino acids, are the essential nitrogen-containing elements in protein that we need. Human life, as we know it, is possible only because protein, available from many food sources, provides the amino acids. That's why all animals, from mice to people, require protein.

Essential Versus Nonessential Amino Acids

All proteins are made from approximately 22 amino acids that are found throughout nature. The amino acids are used to make the protein of body tissues, make hormones, trans-

147

port fat, and make other proteins, such as the enzymes that digest food. Indeed, any body tissue, body function, or body process involves proteins. So it follows that the basic building blocks, the amino acids, are very important.

Think of the amino acids as 22 different beads that can be linked together in any arrangement. Imagine that this string of amino acid beads is a protein. Since there are 22 amino acids and no limit to how they can be arranged in protein, it follows that there's no limit to the types of protein that can exist.

Of the 22 amino acids we get in food, our body can make all but eight. These eight *essential* amino acids determine the quality of a protein. For example, every protein in our body contains some of the *essential* amino acids. If we didn't get enough of one of the *essential* amino acids, our body would be unable to make the proteins it needs and eventually we'd die. The essential amino acids are so important; we simply can't live without them! Nonessential amino acids are also important. They are similarly used for making protein, and the element nitrogen that they provide is also used in many other body chemicals and tissues. For example, nitrogen is essential in the nucleic acids that make up our genetic material. If we get a generous supply of the nonessential amino acids from food, our body doesn't need to use up energy to make them. So, although we can get along without the nonessential amino acids, they're very important in our diet. They help us thrive rather than just survive.

But in fact, we don't eat amino acids, we eat protein. So protein that contains a good balance of all the essential amino acids and the nonessential amino acids is of better quality than protein that doesn't contain this balance. We'll come back to this point shortly, but first consider the obvious question. Why not just eat amino acids?

Why Not Eat Amino Acids?

Actually, we *do* eat amino acids. Protein is digested in our stomach, and is reduced to its amino acids in the small intestine, so they can be absorbed from the small intestine into the blood. They are then used to make the myriad of body proteins and other materials. Some of them a: even used for energy. Thus it's only desirable to bypass the digestive process under special conditions. A physician and dietician are usually involved in these applications.

Sometimes when the digestive system must rest, or is not functioning, a doctor will prescribe an *elemental diet*. These diets, usually specially prepared under very rigorous conditions, provide all the components of food in their elemental form. These components include protein as amino acids or peptides, and fat and carbohydrate as their basic elements (discussed in Chapter Eight). They allow the body to be nourished without the necessity of digestion. In routine cases the diets are taken by mouth; in more advanced cases they are tubed directly into the stomach; and in the most sophisticated diet form, Total Parenteral Nutrition, the elements are pumped directly into the blood. TPN solutions contain the amino acids together with all other nutrients; they require specialized medical supervision at first, but can be personally administered at home.

Satisfying your protein requirement by purchasing pills or powders of amino acids is very costly. And in addition to being expensive, it requires a complex juggling of the amounts of one amino acid versus another. In fact, to do it correctly would require the supervision and practical experience of a registered dietician. Even the average registered dietician would have a tough time planning it; that's why a dietician who specializes in clinical techniques is consulted when it's necessary.

So, you ask, "What about the amino acids we see for sale in health food stores, drugstores, and some supermarkets?" Those amino acids are generally sold for *perceived* rather than *real* needs. They are generally advertised to body builders on the notion that they will supply an extra protein-building capacity. They don't build extra protein capacity and the illusion that they do helps only the people who manufacture them. Although evidence suggests that body builders can get *slightly* better results from their weight lifting if they use lots of protein, the notion that taking pills of amino acids for that purpose totally lacks substance.

The best way to satisfy the body's need for the essential and nonessential amino acid is from protein—protein derived from food in a well-balanced diet.

Protein Quality

Protein quality is determined by the amount of each essential amino acid it contains. The old saying "a chain is as strong as its weakest link" is a good description. The quality of a protein can't be any better than the limiting amount of any one of the essential amino acids. Actually, some proteins are better than others, because the amounts of each of the essential amino acids relative to each other are just right. We say their amino-acid distribution is excellent. Proteins from animals are generally the best quality. Indeed, a system of determining protein quality has been established with cow's milk protein, or casein, as its standard. There's a standard maintained at the National Bureau of Standards for this purpose.

The standard measure for protein quality is determined by how well young newly weaned laboratory rats grow. Because they are already growing rapidly, the protein quality is immediately obvious if the rats' growth rate improves or falters. With rapid growth as a criteria, protein sources can conveniently be graded. The grading system is called PER, which is short for "protein efficiency ratio." Don't let the sophisticated-sounding terms confuse you; it's really quite easy to understand.

If a protein has a PER as good or better than casein, we set the adult requirement for it at 45 grams daily; if it's less than casein, we set the requirement at 65 grams. In everyday terms that means if you weigh about 150 pounds, you should get 45 grams, or just under 2 ounces, of protein that's as good or better than milk protein. Alternatively, the same

150-pound person should get 65 grams, or about 2½ ounces, if the protein quality is less than that of casein.

Protein as Food

Protein in some foods is complete. Eggs, meat, fish, fowl, and dairy products are all sufficient by themselves. If any one of them were your only source of protein, your taste buds might get bored, but nutritionally you'd get along very well, hence the term *complete proteins*.

Some foods provide good protein, but fall short in one or more of the essential amino acids. Since these proteins need to be complemented with other proteins, we call them complementary protein foods. They include grain, nuts, beans, and peas—the legumes. These foods should not serve as the sole source of protein, because they fall short of one or more essential amino acids. And you have to eat a lot of them to get enough protein. That's why nutritionists urge people to eat a variety of foods. Variety is especially important for vegetarians, because vegetable proteins are seldom adequate by themselves and must be "complemented." That's why they're usually called complementary proteins. If you mix beans with rice, the rice makes up the shortcoming of the beans and vice versa. The protein mixture is then complete. Alternatively, eat milk with cereal, or yogurt with beans; the extra essential amino acids in the dairy products will complement the shortfall in the grains or beans. Similarly meat, fish, and fowl complete these complementary proteins. I'm sure you get the idea. Some eggs with very high PER can complement and complete the protein of vegetable meals. In fact, it takes just a small amount of animal protein to complement vegetable protein; for example, a meal of rice with a small amount of chicken or eggs is an excellent source of protein.

Protein in each meal needn't be nutritionally complete. It's an average we're after. Let's say you have cereal or grains for breakfast, some fish or fowl at lunch, and pasta at dinner. You'll get protein from the cereal, grain (pasta), and fish. But most important, the fish at lunch will provide enough essential amino acids to compensate for the shortfall in the pasta and cereal. If you have milk or yogurt with the cereal, you've gained added nutritional insurance. In this case, we could call it protein insurance.

Other foods, such as vegetables and fruits, are not significant sources of protein. We simply rate foods as insignificant sources of protein and recognize that we need them for other equally important purposes; but the small amount of protein they provide contributes to the daily total.

Meat as Condiment

This brief review of protein shows that the best quality protein comes from animal foods and that vegetable protein is often incomplete. How therefore can so much of humanity thrive as vegetarians and not as meat eaters, like North Americans? It's because they use meat and other animal products as *condiments*. A small amount of meat, fish, fowl, egg, cheese, or milk protein (e.g., as yogurt) completes the protein in a meal of beans, rice, legumes, pasta, tofu, and other vegetarian foods. The abundance of essential amino acids in small amounts of animal protein can complement many vegetarian foods.

Think about this the next time you eat a meal with ethnic origins. Excellent examples include Chinese foods, pasta, curry dishes, and even haute French cuisine. Most of these foods developed in countries where meat was scarce, but vegetarian foods flourished. Consequently, people learned to stretch the valuable food resources of meat, milk, and eggs, while getting excellent protein to thrive, not simply survive. They used a lot of creativity.

Protein as Energy

Protein can be used by the body to make energy. The primary energy nutrients are fat and carbohydrate, but protein also serves to some extent. As a source of energy, however, protein is not only inefficient, but expensive. Many reducing diets provide 35 percent of their Calories as protein. This happens because you require 45 to 65 grams of protein daily even if you're dieting. Much of this protein goes for Calories and accelerates weight loss, because of its inefficiency as a Calorie source. If a large excess of protein is eaten, it is used as energy, especially if fat and carbohydrate are in short supply. If there's adequate fat and carbohydrate, with excess protein, then there's a Calorie excess and the body stores it as fat.

Through a complex series of interactions, excess nonessential amino acids are converted to carbohydrate. After a protein-rich meal, people sometimes feel satisfied for a long period—several hours or more. This results from the extra amino acids being converted to carbohydrate and getting used for energy. Eating excess protein is wasteful, however, because it gets used for energy rather than building tissue; carbohydrate and fat are the preferred sources of energy.

Protein Need: Back to the RDA

If protein falls below that of casein in quality, an adult needs 65 grams daily. In contrast, we need only 45 grams if the protein is better in quality than casein. We call these needs the RDA—recommended daily allowance. I've included them on page 375 at the end of this book.

Like all nutrients, our protein needs vary with age. Growing children need more per pound of body weight than an adult. On a body-weight basis, our protein need continually declines to about age 20; after that age it generally remains the same. For example, an infant requires 2.2 grams of protein per kilogram of body weight and an adult requires 0.8 grams per kilogram. To put that in perspective; think of an infant at 100 pounds. The 100-pound infant would require 100 grams of protein, or 3.6 ounces daily. In contrast, a 100-pound adult requires 36 grams—that's only 1.28 ounces. An infant is a small metabolic dynamo because it's growing; in contrast, the adult's metabolism has slowed down to a maintenance level. But since the infant weighs less, it gets along on less total protein. If we fed infants on a per-pound basis, we'd realize that they require enormous amounts of food. But because they're small, the total amount required is relatively low.

A short calculation will give you some idea of your own protein need. I've prepared Table 11.1 to show weight in pounds and kilograms, and the protein requirement in grams and ounces. The list is based on protein close to, but not quite as good as, casein. You can see from this why the 65-gram requirement, expressed on many food labels, strikes a convenient average. If the protein is better than casein in quality, you can get by with less.

TABLE 11.1
Adult
Protein Requirement

Body Weight		Protein Requirement	
Pounds	**Kilograms**	**Grams**	**Ounces**
100	45	36	1.3
120	54	43	1.5
140	64	51	1.8
160	73	58	2.1
180	82	66	2.4
200	91	73	2.6

This tabulation expresses the protein requirement of adults when the protein is of "good" quality but not "excellent," like casein, or other animal protein, such as eggs, meat, or fish.

The Caloric Cost of Protein Sources

Animal protein comes with the energy reserves animals store best—fat. Vegetable protein comes with carbohydrate, because that's how vegetables store energy. So animal protein comes with fat, and vegetable protein comes with carbohydrate. Since protein also provides Calories, the total Caloric delivery of food is a combination of both.

Table 11.2 illustrates how many Calories are required to get an ounce of protein. One ounce is 28 grams of protein, or 43 percent of the recommended daily allowance of 60 grams. Table 11.2 gives insight into the origin of Calories in protein-rich foods. You can also see why adding meat or fish to rice increases the overall protein quality. At the same time, the rice reduces the percent of Calories from fat and increases the Calories from carbohydrate.

TABLE 11.2
An Ounce of Protein
from Various Food Sources
or
The Caloric Costs of an Ounce of Protein

Food	Amount in Ounces	Total Calories	Calories	
			% as Fat	% as Carbohydrate
Oatmeal (dry)	6 (2 cups)	663	16	68
Brick cheese	4.2	445	72	3
Cottage cheese (2% fat)	1.1	225	20	16
Egg	8 (4.6 eggs)	363	64	3
Striped bass	5.6	152	22	None
Salmon	5.0	200	40	None
Clams (large)	8 (10 clams)	161	11	14
Spaghetti	26 (5.4 cups) cooked)	856	4	85

Food	Amount in Ounces	Total Calories	Calories	
			% as Fat	% as Carbohydrate
Lean ground beef	4	285	58	None
Regular ground beef	4.3	349	66	None
Prime rib	4.5	471	75	None
Bacon	3.2	530	77	None
Roast pork	5.7	464	74	None
Cured ham	4.9	289	56	None
Link sausage	11 links (139 oz.)	516	77	None
Beef frankfurter	4 franks (8.3 oz.)	730	81	2
Low-fat 2% milk	28	418	35	39
Low-fat 1% milk protein fortified	23	343	22	46
Lactaid milk (low-fat)	28	357	26	47
Yogurt (low-fat)	21	798	15	71
Yogurt (cream)	22	1032	35	54
Almonds	4.7	821	75	12
Chicken dark meat (no skin)	3.5	205	42	None
Chicken white meat (no skin)	3.2	157	23	None
Turkey white meat (no skin)	3.3	147	18	None
Goose (no skin)	3.4	229	48	None
Beans (baked) (with pork)	2 cups	764	31	57
Black beans (boiled)	1.8 cups	418	4	72

Food	Amount in Ounces	Total Calories	Calories % as Fat	% as Carbohydrate

Same for kidney beans, lima beans, and most other common beans

Food	Amount in Ounces	Total Calories	Fat	Carbohydrate
Mushrooms	46	345	17	76
White rice	51 (7 cups)	1561	None	89
Brown rice	40 (5.7 cups)	1326	5	86

The amount of specific foods required to get 1 ounce of protein; the data are for foods cooked without adding anything; for example, roasting meat, fish, or fowl, and boiling vegetables. The data are adopted from *Bowes and Church's Food Values of Portions Commonly Used*, by Jean A. Pennington (15th edition, 1989, J. B. Lippincott Co.).

Table 11.2 shows that animal foods are the most efficient sources of protein. For example, to get adequate protein from rice would mean a lot of eating as well as many Calories; similarly for most other high-protein vegetables. The most Caloric-efficient protein sources are fish and the white meat of fowl.

Think about how you get sufficient protein in a day. I have tabulated some typical meals by using the information in Table 11.2. You can easily do the same by using a pocket calculator. Table 11.3 shows a simple food pattern that contains 59 grams of protein from fewer than 1,000 Calories, leaving room for other foods and snacks.

In addition to the protein sources in Table 11.3, you need other foods. A daily menu plan should include two pieces of fruit, four vegetables, and one serving of salad. (An apple, pear, orange, or banana each count as one fruit. A serving of vegetables would be spinach, carrots, peas, or corn, to name just a few. The salad should contain some colored vegetables, including lettuce. We discuss this in more detail in Chapter Fourteen.)

TABLE 11.3
A Menu that Provides 90 percent of the RDA in Protein Under 1,000 Calories*

Food	Serving Size	Protein	Calories
Oatmeal	⅓ cup (dry)	5 grams	109
Milk (2% fortified)	½ cup	4	60
Lean hamburger	3.5 oz.	24	268
Rice	1 cup	4	223
Spaghetti	1 cup	5	158
with 6 clams	6	17	97
Totals		59 grams	915 calories

*If other foods are eaten, for example, some breads, vegetables, fruit, and more milk, the 65-gram RDA of protein will be exceeded.

Putting It Together

Protein, essential for life and health, can be obtained from many foods. The most efficient source is animal products, such as the meat of fish, fowl, and animals. Other excellent sources include eggs and dairy products, such as milk, cheese, and yogurt. If protein sources are mixed—for example, rice with fish or spaghetti with clams—the total protein quality is good and the percentage of calories from fat is reduced.

Now we're ready to consider fat. From Table 11.2 you can see that fat is provided by foods of animal origin, but not from foods of vegetable origin. Fat is one of the major concerns for people with any dietary problems. Let's see what we can learn from Table 11.2: 3 ounces of oatmeal with 14 ounces of Lactaid milk (the equivalent of three meals) yields an ounce of protein, with 510 Calories mostly from carbohydrate. Compare that to four frankfurters, with 730 Calories, all from fat. One 5-ounce serving of salmon, with its excellent omega-3 oils, is only 200 Calories, compared to 4.5 ounces of prime rib, at more than twice the Calories, mostly saturated fat and no omega-3 oils. A serving of chicken breast (white meat) with 157 Calories compares to 11 link sausages at 516 Calories, 21 ounces of low-fat yogurt at 798 Calories, or 5.7 ounces of roast pork at 464 Calories.

A meal consisting of 1 ounce of chicken and 4.5 cups of white rice would provide 1,100 Calories, no significant amount of fat, an ounce of protein—and would satisfy most people. I know that 4.5 cups of rice is a lot, but I had to use that much to get the correct amount of protein with only 1 ounce of chicken. Although this is not a typical American dish, it is typical in a country such as Malaysia. Many people do very well on food just like this.

My objective is for you to understand the following: Excellent protein can be obtained from foods that supply a small number of Calories, and an inconsequential amount of these Calories comes from fat.

After thinking about Table 11.2, turn to Table 11.3 in which I've set up a menu to provide 60 grams of protein from fewer than 1,000 Calories. Less than 25 percent of the Calories are from fat. (Notice that I've used spaghetti with clam sauce; my Italian background couldn't remain submerged.) I urge you to experiment on paper, for yourself, to see how you can get 60 grams of protein with little fat and Calories. The other Calories in your diet can be eaten as high-carbohydrate foods that are easily digested and cause no bowel discomfort—for example, brown rice, mashed potatoes, or well-ripened, peeled fruit.

CHAPTER TWELVE

Dietary Fats and Oils

We're all familiar with fat. Most people know intuitively that some foods, like butter, are all fat; other foods, such as bacon and ham, are high in fat and still others, such as white turkey meat, are low in fat. But there's also some confusion; for example, people think that margarine and light oil, such as corn oil, have fewer Calories than butter. They don't. And since most of us are trying to avoid cholesterol, many foods, such as margarine, are advertised as having "no cholesterol" even if they're all fat.

To make things more confusing, nutritionists say that we should strive to get no more than 30 percent of our Calories from fat. They also claim that we should strive for a ratio of polyunsaturated fat to saturated fat of 1:1 with the majority of fat as monounsaturated. So you ask: "What's a polyunsaturated fat, and what's a monounsaturated fat?" And if all that's not enough, evidence is mounting that individuals with IBD should strive for more omega-3 oils in their diet. Don't let that throw you, because I'll sort it all out. But if you feel a little confused, you're not alone.

Saturated Versus Unsaturated Fat

What do a stick of butter, a bottle of olive oil, a stick of margarine, and corn oil have in common? They're all fat and provide 9 Calories per gram. That's 252 Calories per ounce, or 85 Calories per tablespoon. Olive oil is much better for you than the butter, and you should strive for a variety of fats and emphasize olive oil a little more than corn oil.

You're already familiar with the two major groups of fat, saturated and unsaturated, although you might not have thought of them that way. Saturated fat is hard at room temperature and unsaturated fat is liquid at room temperature. Your refrigerator and cupboard probably store some examples of each.

Butter is a fine example of saturated fat. It's solid at room temperature. In fact, that's why we call saturated fat "hard fat." The hard white fat around a piece of beef, pork, or ham is also saturated fat. Though it's harder to see, the fat that marbles an expensive filet of beef is similarly saturated. Animal fat is hard at room temperature and becomes softer at body temperature.

In contrast to saturated fat, unsaturated fat is liquid and usually clear at room temperature. Perhaps you have some vegetable oil, perhaps some corn oil, peanut oil, or olive oil in your cupboard or pantry. All are clear liquids at room temperature. Each of them contains a small amount of saturated fat dissolved in the unsaturated oils. If you have several types, notice that some oils seem lighter than others. If you don't have any safflower oil, look at some the next time you're in the supermarket. Safflower oil is almost water clear. That's because it's mostly polyunsaturated.

You can differentiate fats quickly by asking one question, "Is it liquid or solid at room temperature?" If it's liquid, it's mostly unsaturated, and if it's solid, it's more saturated. By inspection you can tell that some unsaturated oils are lighter than others. You can do another test. Put some oils in the refrigerator. Some become cloudy, whereas others stay clear; the cloudy oils have more saturated fat. Lighter oils are called polyunsaturated—"poly" meaning much.

Saturated (SFA), Monounsaturated (MFA), Polyunsaturated (PUFA)

Chemists tell us that the structure of hard fat is dense and very firm—"highly saturated" is the term they use. There's no open space to add anything further. In contrast, the vegetable oils are not dense and uniform. They contain open spaces so things can be added—"unsaturated" is the term.

The terms *saturated* and *unsaturated* refer specifically to the actual chemical structure or molecular configuration. In a saturated fat (SFA for short) the actual linkages holding the carbon atoms together are all used up. In monounsaturated oils (MFA for short) one linkage is unused; the fat is not quite as dense and uniform. Since "poly" means many, it follows that in polyunsaturated oils (PUFA) many spaces are left open. It's much less dense than either saturated or monounsaturated fat. Now you know the chemistry and are comfortable with the idea that oils are unsaturated and hard fats are saturated. The more unsaturated, the lighter the oil.

Olive oil is an excellent example of MFA. While liquid at room temperature, MFA oils tend to be amber and somewhat thick. These oils flow more slowly, or are "moderately viscous." (*Viscosity* is a technical word that describes flowability. If we say it's highly viscous, it means it doesn't flow easily.)

Sunflower oil is PUFA oil. It's light, very fluid, and much less viscous than olive oil. The more unsaturated these PUFA oils, the clearer and less viscous they become. Safflower, the most unsaturated of all the oils, looks and flows like water.

Beef lard is an SFA. It's solid, even at body temperature; in fact it's white and hard. Most animal fat is this way; the most common examples are beef and pork fat. "Hard fat" is a good description for them.

Omega-3 Versus Omega-6 Oils

Chemists can separate PUFAs even more based on the location of the open or reactive spaces. Counting from one end of the fat molecule, called the omega end of the fat molecule, the reactive center is either six units in, or three units in; so it's called either omega-6 or omega-3. Both are used by our body to make the prostaglandins, some hormonelike materials essential to many body processes. Don't let the word *prostaglandin* throw you, but be aware that two prostaglandins are very important; one is made from omega-6 fatty acids, and one is made from the omega-3 fatty acids.

In North America our diets are rich in the omega-6 oils. It's found in abundance in corn, soy, and sunflower oils, and in animal fat; in short, it's everywhere. In contrast, the omega-3 oils are found in the chloroplasts of green plants, cold-water blue-skinned fish, nuts that grow on trees, and some seeds, such as flax, sesame, and several others. It's not found in domesticated animal fat, but is in the fat of wild forage animals, including deer, elk, moose, rabbit, and a few others most of us don't eat.

We could never eat enough green leafy vegetables to satisfy our need for omega-3 oils. Our best strategy is to get it from cold-water fish. Cold-water, oily fish, like salmon, mackerel, anchovies, and others eat algae that contain lots of the omega-3 oils, or they eat other fish that have eaten the seaweed or algae. From this you can see that the omega-3 oil goes up the food chain to the biggest fish of all. In fish these oils are concentrated, making fish excellent sources of the omega-3 oils. Similarly with foraging animals, such as deer and rabbits.

The omega-6 oil most commonly available in the diet is linoleic acid. It's found in corn oil, soy oil, and most vegetable oils. It's converted to another omega-6 oil, arachidonic acid, in our bodies, and the bodies of all animals. So, we get arachidonic acid, the major omega-6 oil, from all animal foods. Linoleic and arachidonic acids are abundant in our diets.

The omega-3 oil alpha linolenic acid (ALA) is found in green plants and is converted to eicosapentaenoic acid, EPA for short. Our bodies make EPA from ALA, as do most other animals and fish. Fish, however, concentrate EPA in their tissues, so they are the best source. Our foods are rich in the omega-6 oils and contain almost none of the omega-3. Domestic beef and other farm animals are raised on corn and other grains that are devoid of the omega-3 oils but rich in the omega-6 oils. The only way out of the dilemma is to eat fish, oil-containing nuts and seeds, or use the oils from these sources.

Why We Need Omega-3 Oils

Dr. Jorn Dyerberg studied people living in Greenland and their forebears living in Denmark and compared the health of one to the other. Other scientists compared people living in the seacoast villages of Japan to people living inland. People in Greenland and the coastal villages of Japan eat a diet naturally balanced between omega-6 and omega-3. In contrast, people in Denmark and the inland villages of Japan eat a diet that is abundant in the omega-6 oils and almost devoid of the omega-3 oils.

One striking difference in the disease patterns related to these diets was the inflammatory diseases. Folks whose diet is balanced in the omega-6 and omega-3 have a much lower incidence of inflammatory disease. In contrast, most Americans whose diets favor omega-6 oils have lots of inflammatory disease. The inflammatory diseases studied focused on arthritis, psoriasis, asthma, and polyarthritis. The investigators didn't study the inflammatory bowel diseases; there simply wasn't any in the population they studied.

Other scientists have picked up on the findings, however. Research in Denmark at the Bispebjerg Hospital gives us some insight. The bowels of people with IBD are exceptionally rich in prostaglandin made from the omega-6 oils and contain very little of the prostaglandin made from the omega-3 oils.

There can be many interpretations of this Danish research and it will undoubtedly continue into the next century. Indeed, the differences in the prostaglandin levels could be the result of IBD and have nothing to do with its cause. Inflammation is the end result of things gone awry in many body systems, including the immune system, and all of them involve the prostaglandins. The findings so far make the need for some dietary omega-3 oils even more urgent. We know at this early stage in the science that getting more omega-3 oils in the diet can't hurt—and there's a reasonable chance it will do some good.

How Much Omega-3?

Our dietary problems are the omega-3 oils—ALA and EPA—rather than the omega-6 oils linoleic and arachidonic acids. Some scientists argue that we should get 2 to 3 grams of omega-3 oils daily in our diet. While that level seems high to me, half of it, about 1 gram as a target amount, is an achievable target for everyone. It simply means eating fish twice or more times weekly and making more generous use of alternate oils. The oils of choice are nut oils, such as walnut, avocado, Puritan oil, and canola oil. Flax seed oil is excellent and can be used effectively in baking. To strike a better balance between omega-6 and omega-3 oils, reduce the omega-6 and emphasize the monounsaturated fatty oils. Since this sounds like a tall order, let's see where the fat is coming from.

Sources of Dietary Fat

Table 12.1 lists food by the percent of fat. It also gives the composition of SFA, MFA, and PUFA as a percent of the food. The numbers don't always add up to 100 percent because the foods contain traces of other fatty materials. Fats such as butter and oils contain some water and traces of other components. In addition, some information is lost in rounding off. However, Table 12.1 gives the information you need to select food on the basis of its fat content. It will help you select foods that have a modest to low fat composition. For example, if we seek to reduce total fat, especially saturated fat, we'd select lean beef, trimmed pork, and the white meat of fowl and fish. We'll cover this in greater detail later. For now, let's look at the omega-3 and omega-6 oils and see what rules seem to apply.

TABLE 12.1
The Fat Content of Food
Percent by Weight

	Fat	SFA	MFA	PUF	Calorie % Fat
Food					
Milk 3.5%	3.5	2	1.5	None	50
Milk 2%	2	1.2	0.8	—	31
Milk, skim	Trace	—	—		None
Cheese (average)	32	1	11	3	70
Ice Cream (average)	11	6	3	2	49
Yogurt (low-fat)	2	1	1		29
Egg	12	4	6	Trace	67
Beef (regular ground)	20	10	10	—	62

	Fat	SFA	MFA	PUF	Calorie % Fat
Beef (lean)	20	9	9	2	62
Chicken w/o skin	3.5	1	1	1	23
Chicken with skin	6.5	2	3	2	29
Chicken dark	10	3	5	2	40
Lamb (lean)	8	4	3	1	38
Lamb (lean & fat, ground)	29	16	11	2	74
Pork (lean)	13	4	6	3	70
Pork, ground w. fat	29	12	14	3	73
Frankfurter	27	27	—	—	79
Shellfish	2	—	—	—	14
Finfish (oily)	6		3	3	37
Finfish (filet)	5	None	3	2	26
Wheat bread	2		2		10
Chocolate cake with icing	11	4	5	2	27
Danish pastry	22	7	11	4	50
Beans (average)	None	None			None
Butter	81	45	27	3	100
Lard	100	38	46	16	100
Margarine	81	15	41	22	100
Corn oil	100	10	28	53	100
Cottonseed	100	25	21	50	100
Olive	100	11	76	7	100
Peanut	100	18	47	29	100
Safflower	100	8	17	75	100
Soybean	100	15	20	52	100

Tables 12.2 and 12.3 list sources of omega-3 oils and the calorie content of commonly used spreads and oils. This information, along with Table 12.1, can be used to increase consumption of omega-3 oils and reduce total fat.

TABLE 12.2
Sources of Omega-3 Oils

Food	Omega-3 Content
	Grams per 3½ Ounce Serving
Salmon	1 to 2.5
Mackerel	0.7 to 2.5
Anchovy	0.7 to 1.5
Cod	0.3
Striped bass	0.2 to 0.8
Snapper	0.1 to 0.3
Shellfish	0.5
Trout	0.2 to 1.0
Tuna	0.4 to 2.5

Oils That Provide Omega-3 Oils

Walnut	Rapeseed
Flax seed	Avocado
Sesame seed	Puritan oil
Soybean	Canola oil
Cod-liver oil	
Salmon oil	
Menhaden oil	

TABLE 12.3
Calorie Content of Commonly Used Spreads and Oils per Tablepoon

Spreads	Calories
Butter	108
Whipped butter	81
Butter Buds (1-T. liquid)	6
Margarine (all sources)	100
Whipped margarine (all sources)	70
Diet margarine (low-calorie)	50
Mayonnaise	100
Low-calorie mayonnaise	35
Vegetable oil spreads	80
50% oil	80

Fish Oil Supplements in IBD

Shortly after Dr. Jorn Dyerberg's research about the Greenlanders and Danes was published, fish-oil supplements began to appear in health food stores. One of the earliest forms of food supplements was the daily spoonful of cod-liver oil. Fish-oil supplements aren't really new; it's just that the new ones are rich in EPA and not the vitamins A and D, which were the original selling components of cod-liver oil.

Dyerberg's findings, and subsequent worldwide research has shown clearly that the omega-3 oils, specifically EPA, play an important role in health. In fact, much of the research was conducted with EPA or marine lipid supplements. Most researchers emphasized the benefits of these oils on cardiovascular diseases and high blood pressure. Other researchers focused on the inflammatory diseases, such as arthritis and psoriasis. Furthermore, the researchers could give the volunteers large, daily supplements of EPA because they were in a clinical environment. None of the research emphasized IBD; therefore, although the research in Denmark suggests that such supplements could be beneficial, it's unproven at this time. Suffice to say that at this early stage we know it can't hurt.

It's impractical and possibly even unsafe to use supplements on your own to get the large amounts of EPA used in research. If you don't eat fish and want to insure that you get some EPA and the other omega-3 oils, however, sensible supplementation of about ½ to 1 gram each day is acceptable. That's one or two capsules daily. For the average person who seeks to get it from food, it's about one 3-ounce serving of salmon daily.

Put more simply, you've got to eat, and fish is just about as good as food can get. For example, Table 11.2 shows clearly that it is the most efficient source of high-quality protein.

Cholesterol

Cholesterol is one of the buzz words of our society. Blood cholesterol is used as a simple index of the state of sludge deposited on the walls of our cardiovascular system. As our blood cholesterol goes up, so does the sludge, called plaque, that gets deposited on the walls of our arteries. Among other things, plaque consists of cholesterol. It follows that we want to lower blood cholesterol.

Lowering cholesterol, or not letting it rise in the first place, means following four simple dietary rules:

1. Keep dietary cholesterol below 250 mg. daily.
2. Eat a moderately low-fat diet and increase the ratio of PUFA to SFA.
3. Eat a high-fiber diet of 30 grams or more daily. (Fiber is discussed in chapters Five and Fourteen.)
4. Maintain ideal weight. (This isn't a problem in IBD, but do see Chapter Twenty-Four.)

Cholesterol is an animal product. Our body produces plenty of it because it's necessary. Conversely, there simply isn't any cholesterol in vegetable foods. So a margarine advertisement that says "No cholesterol" is like saying "Water is wet." It follows that we get cholesterol when we eat meat, dairy products, fish, or the flesh from anything that is not from the plant kingdom.

However, the major dietary sources of cholesterol are organ and high fat meats. Look again at Table 12.1. As the percentage of saturated fat increases in animal food, so does the cholesterol content. Select low-fat meat, emphasize white meat of fowl, and eat lots of fish. If you do, you'll keep your fat below 30 percent of calories and your cholesterol to less than 150 milligrams daily.

Before I leave the discussion of cholesterol I must touch on the much-maligned egg. Eggs are good food! They provide the very best quality protein nature has to offer. And for the protein you get, eggs are inexpensive! In addition, eggs contain natural chemicals that help to lower blood cholesterol. The egg has simply gotten bad press; used in moderation, they're just about the best source of protein available in the supermarket. And the versatility of eggs in cooking is almost legend. But one large egg contains about 200 milligrams of cholesterol. If you don't eat two eggs at a sitting, you're in an excellent position.

Lecithin

Lecithin is a naturally occurring fat that is found in oil-bearing plants, egg yolks, and some animal fats. Lecithin has been credited with accomplishing everything from cholesterol reduction to improving mental abilities, so it seems worthwhile to discuss just what lecithin *does* accomplish.

Lecithin consists of three major fatty substances: choline, inositol, and linoleic acid. You've already encountered linoleic acid. It's the major omega-6 PUFA found in plants. It has a moderate cholesterol-lowering ability. Choline and inositol are important for the function of our nervous system. At one time some scientists proposed that they be given the status of B vitamins, but this proposal was dropped. But the notion that they are vitamins still persists, and you sometimes see them listed with vitamin preparations. Indeed, research has shown that they aid mental and nervous system function under some specialized conditions. The research was conducted using lecithin supplements. Even though it was done on lecithin supplements that aren't available to the public, that never seemed to matter. Hence the conclusion that lecithin supplements improve mental acuity.

One rumor is that lecithin will dissolve fat, specifically cellulite. That's nonsense. Lecithin is an emulsifier, but it has no effect on body fat. In fact, one could argue that using large amounts of lecithin could add to your fat, because it provides Calories.

Should you use supplemental lecithin? I believe that our food provides all the lecithin we need. A person with IBD should use sensible food supplements that help provide a good balance of vitamins, minerals, and fiber. Further, if you don't eat fish, the money would be much more wisely spent on one or two capsules of EPA daily.

Calories

Fats and oils in any form provide 9 Calories per gram. No matter how important the product sounds, the Calorie delivery is the same. The commonly used units of measure are listed in Table 12.4.

TABLE 12.4
Fat Calories in Some
Common Units of Measure
Weight

Unit	Calories
Gram	9
Ounce (28.35 grams)	255
Pound (454 grams)	4086

Volume

Teaspoon (4.9 ml, about 4.9 grams)	44
Tablespoon (3 teaspoons)	133
1 fluid ounce (2 tablespoons)	266
1 cup (8 fluid ounces)	2129

Whenever you put a 1-ounce pat of butter on a baked potato, stop and think about this: A baked potato provides about 200 Calories depending on size; 1 ounce of butter or margarine adds 255 Calories. Put another way, the condiment contributes more Calories than the food! I enjoy the surprised expressions on people's faces after they're told potatoes are not fattening and I take them through that explanation. They usually start using sour cream, which has half the Calories of butter.

What about low-Calorie spreads? All spreads contain varying levels of fat. Some contain water; some are whipped and contain air; still others are blended with starch and contain fewer calories. I've listed some commonly used spreads to give you a feeling for the Calories per serving.

From Table 12.3 you can see that most spreads that look, act, and taste like butter deliver about 100 Calories per tablespoon. Whipping and reducing the oil or fat by about 50 percent reduces Calories to about 50 per tablespoon. Butter Buds are a truly low-Calorie substitute for butter.

Get Good Fat Balance: Putting It All Together

Fat is one of the most important and least understood parts of our diet. Now that we've explored the types of dietary fat that we get from food, we'll learn how we should put them together in a good diet. First a few rules.

Rule 1: Keep fat to fewer than 30 percent of calories.
Rule 2: Maintain a ratio of PUFA to SFA of one.
Rule 3: PUFA should provide about 6 percent of calories.
Rule 4: Keep cholesterol intake below about 300 mg daily.

We'll discuss carbohydrates in the next chapter, but at this point we can already plan a diet that delivers plenty of protein and only 30 percent of Calories from fat. I'll give you some do's and don'ts that work.

Dietary Do's

Do: have at least one meal besides breakfast with no meat every day.

Do: eat red meat only twice weekly

Do: select white meat from fish or poultry.

Do: eat an egg twice weekly—but no red meat on the same day.

Do: one completely meatless day each week, including fish, fowl, and four-legged animals.

Do: use oils for cooking.

Do: use spreads sparingly.

Do: eat fish twice weekly, broiled when possible.

Do: use alternatives to butter, such as sour cream on potatoes.

Do: select low-fat dairy products.

Don't

Don't: eat processed meats.

Don't: eat cheese on a day when eating meat.

Don't: eat organ meats.

Don't: eat the fat on meat or the skin on fowl.

Don't: use butter on meatless days.

Don't: eat eggs more than twice weekly.

Don't: eat sausage, bacon, or eggs without cereal; never eat them on a day with meat.

Don't: cook food in butter, lard, or other saturated fat.

Don't: use whole milk; especially whole homogenized milk.

Summary

Dietary fat provides 9 Calories per gram, 225 per ounce.

We should strive to consume no more than 30 percent of our Calories as fat. Polyunsaturated and monounsaturated fats are better than saturated fat. Strive to eat foods with a good level of the omega-3 polyunsaturated oils, obtained from fish, nuts that grow on trees, and seeds, such as flax and sesame. There's growing evidence that we all need more of these oils in our diet.

CHAPTER THIRTEEN

Carbohydrates:
An Ideal Fuel

Carbohydrates such as starch, fiber, and natural sugars in fruits and vegetables, are the ideal fuel for most body functions and are important to health. But processed and manufactured foods high in sugar are, at least, questionable and, at worse, bad for you. You might not be able to eat one natural sugar—lactose, the milk sugar. Similarly, you might be sensitive to the sugar alcohols, such as sorbitol and xylitol.

What Are Carbohydrates?

Carbohydrates, as the name suggests, contain carbon and "hydrate" (hydrogen and oxygen), the elements of water. If you analyzed any carbohydrate, you'd find carbon, oxygen, and hydrogen. But if your analysis went one step further, you'd find that just about all natural carbohydrates contain one of two simple sugars, glucose or fructose, which have a common origin.

Photosynthesis and Glucose and Fructose

Photosynthesis is the process by which a green plant uses sunlight to extract carbon dioxide from the air or water and combines it with water to make the simple sugar, glucose. This exceedingly complex process is common to all green plants and is the major source of energy on our planet. That's why glucose is so widely distributed in nature. It's the sugar we have circulating in our blood; even our brain uses it for energy.

Plants and most living things can rearrange the structure of glucose slightly to make fructose. This explains why fructose is as widely distributed as glucose, but in somewhat lesser quantity. We call glucose and fructose simple sugars. Scientifically they're "monosaccharides" because they're single units; "mono" means one. And they're sweet; hence "saccharide."

Glucose and fructose are often linked together by plants to make a disaccharide, the double sugar called sucrose. Sucrose occurs widely in nature and is highly concentrated in some plants, such as sugar cane and sugar beets, making it easy to refine and sell as table sugar. Table sugar is the purest and least expensive organic chemical available worldwide. Two glucose units are often arranged into another disaccharide, called maltose. Maltose is found in seeds, especially germinating seeds. Hence, we find maltose in barley, wheat, and other seed grains.

Galactose is another simple sugar, similar in total carbon content to glucose, but with the carbon, hydrogen, and oxygen arranged somewhat differently. It's the only sugar made exclusively by animals. Galactose is never found by itself and is always linked with glucose to form lactose, a common disaccharide. Lactose is found in milk from cows, goats, humans, and all other mammals. Lactose is the carbohydrate source in milk. We'll discuss lactose in more detail later.

Sugar Alcohols (a Diversion)

Plants can change glucose to a number of other simple sugars that are found in small quantities and are generally unimportant. These include xylose, pentose, sedoheptulose, and others. However, some of the sugars are converted in the plant, or by manufacturing companies, into sugar alcohols. Two are important because they're sweet and they are widely used. They are sorbitol and xylitol, made from sucrose and xylose, respectively. Some people can't tolerate them (an issue we'll cover later).

Sweetness

We are born with the ability to detect sweet, sour, salty, and bitter tastes. This ability helps us survive. Thousands of years ago it was important, and it's useful even now. In nature, sweet things provide energy and are generally safe; sour-tasting things are usually spoiled and can contain harmful germs; bitter foods often contain toxic substances; and drinking salt water can kill anyone, especially an infant. The ability to detect sweetness was even acknowledged in Military Survival School, where we were taught to eat sweet things and avoid bitter things when lost behind enemy lines.

Fructose is the sweetest sugar in nature. It's what makes fruits, berries, and some vegetables sweet. Next in sweetness after fructose comes sucrose, table sugar, which gets its sweetness from the fructose it contains, rather than its glucose. Glucose is only about half as sweet as fructose. Xylitol, a sugar alcohol, is about as sweet as sucrose.

Table 13.1 summarizes the sweetness of the most common sugars. By inspection, you can see that after fructose and sucrose, there's no contest.

TABLE 13.1
Relative Sweetness of Common Sugars

Sugar	Relative Sweetness
Fructose	1.0
Sucrose	0.8
Glucose	0.6
Maltose	0.3
Lactose	0.2

Sugar Alcohols

Xylitol	0.8
Sorbitol	0.4

Complex Carbohydrates: Starches

Visualize each sugar as a link with occasional branches. Glucose, fructose, and maltose, a disaccharide, can be linked together in almost endless chains. These chains of simple sugars are called complex carbohydrates, or starches. In this case, "complex" simply means large.

Starch is stored by plants as an energy source. That's why potatoes, rice, wheat, corn, turnips, beans, cereals, grains, and vegetables are starchy. They represent the storage of energy for reproduction. Once people discovered the food value of starch about 10,000 years ago, they started to cultivate starch-containing plants. This led to farming of the major grains, cereals, and tubors, such as potatoes.

You might ask: "Why isn't an apple or pear starchy?" Apples, pears, cherries, and the seeds of most fruit do contain starch, but in the seeds or pits, which we don't eat. For the seeds to be spread, and the species to survive, they rely on animals, even humans, to eat the fruit and either spit out the seeds or pass them in stools. Apples and other fruits are sweet to entice animals to eat them and spread the seed.

Dietary Fiber

Some glucose and maltose are made into carbohydrate materials that aren't digested by humans. These include cellulose, pectin, and a few other materials. We group them together in a class of complex carbohydrates called dietary fiber. Dietary fiber is plant carbohydrate material that isn't digested. Dietary fiber is so important that I've devoted an entire chapter to the subject. But we need to discuss it here briefly so you can see how it relates to carbohydrate metabolism.

Plant cells are protected by a cell wall that's made of tough, coarse fibers called cellulose. These cells are bound together with other nondigestible materials such as lignins, mucilage, pectins, and others. These materials are used to give the plant its shape, protect fruit from drying out, hold parts of it together, and to bind water. Not surprising, they appear in many forms to serve many purposes. For humans, they have one thing in common: they aren't digested. They pass through our stomach and small intestine without breaking down, although some fiber is broken down by bacteria that inhabit the large intestine.

Blood Glucose and Glycogen

Since glucose is the most ubiquitous sugar in nature, it's obvious that all animals, including humans, use it as the most readily available source of energy: carbohydrates provide 4 Calories per gram or 113 grams per ounce.

Our blood contains, on average, 80 to 100 milligrams of glucose per 100 mililiters. (We call it 80 to 100 milligram percent, meaning that it's the milligrams of glucose per 100 milliliters (a deciliter) of blood expressed as percent.) We'll talk more about blood glucose later, but for now, recognize that it's the major source of energy for everything we do.

For instance, it's almost the only source of energy for our brain!

We store energy for two purposes: for short-term use, measured in hours, and long-term, for prolonged activity and against food deprivation for days or weeks. For the short term we rely on carbohydrates, and for the long term we rely on fat. Not surprising, we humans store glucose in our tissues as a type of starch for short-term use; we call this animal starch glycogen.

Glycogen is similar to potato, corn, rice, and other starches. But similar doesn't mean the same. In contrast to starch, glycogen is not a long chain of glucose; it's more like a netting of glucose. This netting doesn't have to supply one unit of glucose at a time; it can allow the chain to release glucose at many points. Therefore, in contrast to starch, glycogen can release a lot of glucose all at once. This is important in times of emergency. For example, in a dangerous situation, our body releases glucose from glycogen very rapidly, pouring a reserve of quick energy into our blood and muscles where it can serve all the organs that need it to help us survive. Glycogen is an effective store of reserve energy that becomes available almost instantly.

Glycogen is stored in our muscles, liver, organs, such as the kidneys, to be used as required. When our blood glucose starts to fall, glycogen is mobilized to release glucose. When we're exercising actively, glycogen is mobilized to keep our blood glucose up. When glycogen's been depleted, such as during a long period of activity, a starchy meal provides raw material, glucose, to restore our glycogen reserves. That's why marathon runners train with large amounts of carbohydrate meals to build glycogen reserves.

Carbohydrate as Energy

By now you know that carbohydrate provides 4 Calories per gram. That's a little less than half of the Calories of fat. This is because carbohydrates are halfway to the end products of energy production—in physiological terms, they're about half-metabolized.

When carbon materials are burned to yield energy, two chemical by-products are given off: carbon dioxide and water. In addition to the carbon, oxygen is used for the combustion. So when we completely burn gasoline, fat, paper, wood, or sugar, carbon dioxide and water are the only by-products, besides the energy that we get as heat. It's no different in our body; when fat or carbohydrate are used, water and carbon dioxide are the by-products, together with the energy. The energy is trapped in other substances and our body heat remains at 98.6° F, since we don't light up!

Now recall that carbohydrate already contains water; hence its name. Fat, in contrast, contains no water. Fat is only carbon and hydrogen. In contrast to carbohydrate, fat hasn't even begun the process.

For this reason, carbohydrate is more easily and more quickly metabolized to produce energy than fat. It requires only half the oxygen. Therefore, for short periods, carbohydrate, specifically glucose, is used for energy because it's the best source. When the need is longer-term, the body mobilizes its fat reserves and starts using them. This is easily seen by comparing the body's requirements for a short run of a half-mile to that of a three-mile run.

An average jogger can run a half-mile in about 5 minutes. The body can supply the energy with its blood glucose; there's not even a need to mobilize glycogen. The three-mile run, in contrast, will take the same person 25 minutes. After the first 5 minutes the body mobilizes its glycogen, and by 10 minutes, it's starting to use some of the circulating blood fats. After 15 minutes, as much as 50 percent of the energy for running comes from fat, and our fat reserves have begun being called into action.

Digestion of Carbohydrate

In the Preface we reviewed the parts of the digestive system. I observed that digestion begins in the mouth with chewing and lubrication. Carbohydrate digestion begins very actively in the mouth. Our saliva, in addition to moistening and lubricating food, contains an enzyme that breaks down starch. You can prove this for yourself by chewing a soda cracker for a long time; you'll notice how it starts out bland, but begins to taste sweet. The starch in soda crackers breaks down in our mouth to maltose.

Starches are not digested in the stomach, but once in the small intestine they're completely broken down to glucose. Sucrose is split by sucrase to glucose, and fructose and lactose is split by lactase to glucose and galactose. (Many people, especially those with intestinal disorders, and some ethnic groups who lack the enzyme lactase, cannot digest lactose. This problem is so important for folks with IBD that I have devoted Chapter Four, entitled "Symptoms of Lactose Intolerance," to the subject.)

Absorption of Sugar

We don't absorb starch into our blood; we absorb the simple sugars glucose, fructose, and galactose. A few other minor sugars and sugar alcohols from vegetables and fruits are similarly absorbed.

Absorption of glucose from starch takes place as the starch is broken down. Remember, starch is like a long chain with few branches and digestion proceeds from the ends. It follows then that glucose is released more slowly from starch than from the disaccharide, sucrose. Nutritionists urge people to eat a diet rich in complex carbohydrates because their breakdown takes time and they're released into the blood slowly.

When you eat a manufactured food, or drink a beverage

that's rich in monosaccharides or in sucrose, the glucose is instantly ready for absorption. Since the intestine is well equipped to absorb glucose, the glucose load crosses the intestine into the blood very quickly. This sugar load signals the body to produce the hormone insulin, which is required for glucose in the blood to cross the cell membranes and be used for energy by the cell.

A heavy sugar load first elevates blood sugar; the body responds by releasing a surge of insulin. Often the insulin is excessive and glucose quickly enters the body cells. The blood sugar drops quickly, producing low-blood sugar, or hypoglycemia. ("Hypo" means low and "glycemia" means sugar; low-blood sugar.) You know from the previous sections that the body strives to maintain stable blood sugar; that's why high-sugar foods should be eaten in moderation.

Fiber in Absorption

Fiber plays an important role in the absorption of glucose. Some scientists did an experiment that is worth describing because it tells the fiber story very nicely.

The scientists used apples prepared in three ways: raw, pureed into an opaque juice with lots of pulp, and as a clarified juice made by filtering the puree. Each preparation was adjusted so it provided the same amount of glucose and fructose as the apple. They had volunteers eat each substance after an overnight fast. On each of three successive days the volunteers received a different preparation.

The apple, as the baseline, changed the blood sugar very little even though all the glucose and fructose from the apple was absorbed. The heavy puree raised blood sugar moderately, about 10 percent from its fasting level. In contrast to both, the clarified juice elevated the blood glucose by more than 20 percent. In each case insulin production was in proportion to the blood sugar change. Consequently, about 90 minutes after drinking the highly clarified puree, the volunteers had low-blood sugar and hypoglycemia, and they were hungry. The only difference in this experiment was the fiber. The apple presented a matrix that consisted of fiber, especially pectin and cellulose. Although the matrix was destroyed in the thick puree, most of the fiber was still present. In the clarified juice there was no fiber.

From experiments like this we say that fiber modulates the absorption of sugar. Actually, it modulates the absorption of fat and amino acids as well, but it's most important in the absorption of glucose and fructose. Therefore, fiber is an essential component in carbohydrate digestion and absorption even though it is not digested itself.

Protein and Carbohydrate Absorption

Protein-rich food also helps to modulate glucose and fructose absorption. This is because protein provides a matrix in the intestine and is digested slowly. Consequently, a protein-rich meal that contains sugar-rich foods modulates sugar absorption. As a result, desserts following a meal do not produce the same sugar "surge" in the blood if they are eaten on an empty stomach.

Selecting Carbohydrate-Rich Foods

Eat natural foods, or processed forms of starch-rich foods! Food selections should emphasize fruits, vegetables, cereals, and grains. When selecting processed foods, choose pasta, cereals such as shredded wheat, whole-grain breads, and foods made with whole potatoes and rice. The apple experiment teaches that juices made from whole fruit should be selected.

Let's look at the carbohydrate content of some natural foods to get a feeling for the percentage of Calories from carbohydrates. I've summarized this analysis in Table 13.2. As you can see, most vegetables and fruits are principally carbohydrates. More than 70 percent of their Calories come from carbohydrates, on average. Some, such as oranges, are almost all carbohydrate. Nuts and avocados are exceptions, because their Calories are largely derived from the oils they contain.

TABLE 13.2
Carbohydrate-Rich Foods

Food	Serving Size	Grams Carbohydrate	Calories	Carbohydrates as Percent Total Calories
Milk (2%)	1 cup	15	60	41
Yogurt	1 cup	13	52	42
Cheese	1 oz	Trace	None	None
Nuts (average)	cup	28	96	11
Beans and peas	cup	38	152	72
Asparagus	cup	5	20	67
Broccoli	cup	7	28	70
Cauliflower	cup	5	20	80
Potato, baked (no skin)	1 potato	21	84	93
Potato, boiled (no skin)	1 potato	23	92	87
Tomato	cup	10	40	80
Avocado	one	13	52	14
Banana	one	26	104	100
Grapefruit	½	12	48	100
Orange	one	16	64	100
Apple	one	18	72	85
Apricots	three	14	56	100
Raspberries	1 cup	17	68	97
Bagel	one	30	120	73
French bread	pound loaf	251	1004	76

Food	Serving Size	Grams Carbohydrate	Calories	Carbohydrates as Percent Total Calories
Rye bread	slice	13	72	87
White	slice	10	40	73
Whole wheat	slice	14	56	86
Cake with chocolate icing	piece	45	180	72
Spaghetti (cooked)	cup	32	128	83
Shredded wheat	1 biscuit	20	80	88

Low-fat milk and yogurt provide about 42 percent of Calories from carbohydrate and most of the remainder from protein. Cheese does not follow this pattern; it provides most of its Calories from fat. Breads and other foods made from grains provide about 70 percent or more of their Calories from carbohydrate.

From this analysis, you can get a feeling for carbohydrates as a percentage of the calories of most natural foods. But this leaves packaged and processed foods. You might ask, what about pizza? Breakfast cereals? How do you know which fruit juice to select? This requires label reading and we'll deal with that next.

Label Reading for Carbohydrates

The nutritional panel on most products provides a complete breakdown of carbohydrates. The top of the nutrition panel lists total carbohydrate content per serving. Multiply this number by 4 to get the total Calories from carbohydrate, divide it into total Calories, and multiply by 100 to get the percentage of Calories from carbohydrate. Then, look at the bottom of the panel under *Carbohydrate Infor-*

mation, which gives the breakdown of starch and related carbohydrates, and sucrose and other sugars, if they are present. Let's look at the ingredient list.

Ingredient List

On the same panel that contains nutritional information is an ingredient list. The nutritional information is not required by law, but the ingredient list is. It is expressed in descending order by weight of the ingredients used to make the product. We'll use Product 19 as an example of a readily available breakfast cereal.

Ingredients reads: corn, oat and wheat flour, sugar, rice, salt, defatted wheat germ, corn syrup, malt flavoring, annatto color. Then the product includes a listing of added vitamins and minerals, which we'll discuss in chapters Sixteen and Seventeen. Product 19's ingredient list tells you that this product is mostly starch. It contains two sources of sugar: sugar, meaning sucrose or table sugar, and corn syrup, which is mostly glucose and fructose.

From the ingredient list and nutrition label of Product 19 you can conclude that the product is mostly starch, with very little whole grain, because 20 of the 24 grams of carbohydrate—that's 83 percent—is starch. Another 13 percent is sugar, so that leaves little room for fiber. A cereal that provides fewer than 3 grams of fiber per serving is not a whole-grain cereal!

The uppermost part of the nutrition panel states that the cereal provides 24 grams of carbohydrate per serving. Four times 24, divided into 100 (total Calories per serving) and multiplied by 100 tells you that 96 percent of the calories in this product come from carbohydrates.

Now look at the bottom of the panel under *Carbohydrate Information*. First, it tells you that starch and related carbohydrates are 20 grams; that means 20 of 24 grams of complex carbohydrate. Next it states that it contains 3 grams of sucrose and other sugars; that means that about 13 percent of the carbohydrate is simple sugar. Product 19 provides 1 gram of fiber. When you read the chapter on fiber, you'll see that 1 gram per serving is not enough. This product doesn't meet my standards for a breakfast cereal.

Two comparisons to Product 19 are Nabisco Shredded Wheat and Quaker Oats. I'll leave their nutritional panel for you to read the next time you're in the supermarket, and we'll deal with them again in Chapter Fourteen.

Nabisco Shredded Wheat has a simple ingredient list. Ingredients: 100% natural whole wheat. It's clean—no sugar, no oils, nothing added. Quaker Oats is a cooked cereal that provides an ideal type of fiber for everybody, especially folks with bowel disorders. It is an elegantly simple cereal. Ingredients: 100% natural rolled oats. I recommend you prepare it without salt.

I'll give you one last comparison: the ingredients list for Cap'n Crunch. It speaks for itself; the product is flour and white and brown sugar with sprayed-on vitamins, some of which are used in lesser quantity than the artificial color on the product:

Ingredients: Corn flour, sugar, oat flour, coconut oil, brown sugar, salt, niacinamide (one of the B vitamins), reduced iron, yellow 5, calcium pantothenate (one of the B vitamins), zinc oxide (a source of zinc), yellow 6, pyridoxine hydrochloride (one of the B vitamins), thiamin mononitrate, BHA (a preservative), riboflavin, folic acid, vitamin B_1.

The lesson here is that sugar is sugar whether it's white or brown. Since corn flour contains some sugar, this product probably contains more sugar than any other ingredient. Another red flag is its sixth ingredient, salt, which we'll discuss in subsequent chapters.

Juice

I picked two fruit juices, both purchased in our local Safeway, for which we only need to read the ingredient list. The nutritional panel will tell you that they provide all their calories from carbohydrates and all the carbohydrates are in the form of simple sugar. However, the ingredient list can be very revealing.

Hawaiian Punch
Ingredients: HP water, corn syrup and sugar, fruit juices and purees, concentrated pineapple, passion fruit, orange and grapefruit juices, apricot, papaya and guava purees, citric acid (provides tartness), natural flavors, vitamin C, dextrin (a flavor carrier), artificial color, artificial flavor, ethyl maltol (a flavor enhancer).

Tiaman's Original Apple Juice
Ingredients: Made from Anderson Valley's finest apples; all natural—no additives, no concentrates.

Hawaiian Punch is mostly water; the HP simply means it's highly purified. That's good. The next two ingredients are sugar. Corn syrup is sugar, and added to sugar it makes this product mostly water and sugar. After that comes a number of fruit concentrates, followed by flavors and flavor enhancers. Since artificial and natural flavors have been added, it's obvious that the juice extracts aren't strong enough to flavor the sugar water.

Hawaiian Punch is actually artificially flavored and colored sugar-water. Do you want to put this into your body? In comparison, the Tiaman's Apple Juice is simply apple juice. It's cloudy, so it's got apple pulp. The pulp settles to some extent, so it needs to be shaken before used. But it's quite close to an apple puree. It's a good product and makes an excellent beverage.

From the ingredient list and the nutritional label you can learn much about the source and type of carbohydrates in packaged food. More than that, the ingredient list tells you how a product has been made. Using both panels regularly and correctly can help you make wise food selections. A good question to ask yourself after analyzing both lists is: "Do I want to put these ingredients into my body?"

Do's for Carbohydrates

Carbohydrate-rich foods should make up about 50 to 60 percent of Calories in your regular diet. However, selection should emphasize foods rich in complex carbohydrate and not simple sugar, with exception of fruit, which is naturally balanced with a fiber content that modulates its sugar absorption.

Do's

Do: eat at least one serving of whole-grain cereal each day. Become familiar with fiber (Chapters Five and Fourteen) so you select ones that don't irritate your intestinal tract.

Do: eat at least two pieces of whole fruit, such as an apple, pear, banana, or three apricots, or alternatively, a full cup of berries, if they do not cause intestinal irritation. Fruit should be peeled; canned fruit can also be used.

Do: eat at least two servings of vegetables, such as asparagus, broccoli, spinach, or brussels sprouts.

Do: eat at least one serving daily of a starchy vegetable, such as potatoes, rice, squash, or pasta.

Do: eat one serving of some beans or other legumes. These include kidney, pinto, navy or lima beans, to name only a few.

Do: eat one serving of salad, with generous green leafy vegetables, and aim for a colored vegetable such as red peppers, tomatoes, or carrots.

Do: eat at least one serving of whole-grain bread, including wheat, rye, or another type, such as oat bread.

Do: drink fruit juice that is made from natural fruit and is, at most, partially clarified. Read the ingredient list.

Don'ts

Don't: eat packaged foods in which sugar is listed as one of the first three ingredients.

Don't: drink juices that contain sugar or corn syrup, especially those with both.

Don't: select breakfast cereals that provide fewer than 3 grams of dietary fiber in a one-cup serving.

Don't: drink more than one serving of sugar-containing soft drinks daily.

Don't: use spreads that contain sugar except for a condiment, such as catsup and mustard.

Don't: use sugar except for a fiber-rich food, such as cereal or as an accompaniment to a fiber-rich meal, such as in a cup of tea or coffee.

Summary

Carbohydrates are essential for health. Indeed, the most widely distributed sugar, glucose, is used by our body as a primary energy source. It can be obtained as starch in vegetables, grains, and some processed foods, such as pasta. A second widely distributed sugar, fructose, imparts sweetness to fruits, even to some vegetables. It's also obtained in sucrose, common table sugar.

The best way to get carbohydrate is in vegetables and fruit because these sources naturally modulate its entry into the bloodstream. This helps to maintain normal blood sugar levels.

Our body contains an excellent carbohydrate reserve, glycogen. Glycogen is a highly branched starch that can be mobilized instantly to maintain normal blood sugar and supply energy for emergencies. A diet with 55 to 65 percent of its Calories from carbohydrate is recommended and will help to maintain excellent glycogen reserves.

CHAPTER FOURTEEN

A Primer on Dietary Fiber: An Apple a Day

An old folk saying is "An apple a day keeps the doctor away." This old English saying, besides selling apples, was good advice. An apple is not a very good source of protein, vitamins, and minerals, but it does provide dietary fiber. Sufficient dietary fiber promotes regularity and helps prevent a number of intestinal disorders. Therefore, the advice, like most folk wisdom, is solid.

Dietary Fiber: Nature's Regulator

Dietary fiber is essential for good bowel regularity and stool consistency. Fiber works both ways. It helps people who too frequently have soft, watery stools to produce stools less frequently and have firmer, more consistent stools. It also helps those with small, hard stools to have more frequent movements with larger stools of softer consistency. This is why I like to call it "nature's regulator." If you're getting enough of the right kind of fiber, your stools should come regularly, move easily, and be consistent. Let's learn more about fiber to see how it can help people with IBD.

What Is Dietary Fiber?

Dietary fiber is the material in plant food that remains undigested after passing through the stomach and small intestine. Just as there are many kinds of fruits, vegetables, grains, and cereals, there are many kinds of dietary fiber. The types of fiber are derived from the role they play in the plant. Some fiber protects the seed and the stem from environmental damage; that's cellulose—it's hard and tough. Some fiber simply holds the plant cells together—that's mucilage. It's like glue. These are the two extreme types of fiber, and there are other types of fiber in between. Each type has properties that are beneficial to health.

Fiber Matrix

A plant cell wall is a fibrous matrix of six different types of fiber. In fact, plant cells are held together in an intact tissue that is a large, continuous fibrous matrix. Some examples of a fibrous matrix are the skins of fruit, such as apples and grapes, the fibrous stems of plants, like asparagus, and the coating on beans. The plant fiber matrix is often overlooked when we focus attention on specific types of fiber.

This fibrous matrix can be exceptionally tough and can remain intact through the entire digestive system. For example, the seed coats of fruits, such as apples and berries, are so tough they pass through the digestive system of animals and birds—that's how nature spreads them from one location to another. It's why human stools often contain seeds, pieces of apple skins, lettuce leaves, chunks of apple, bits of nuts, and other pieces of plant food. Because the matrix is especially tough in many fruits and vegetables, it can be particularly troublesome for people with IBD. That's why I have devoted Chapter Five to a discussion of fiber for people with IBD.

The fiber matrix is more than seed coats and fruit peels. Some partially processed fiber, such as hard wheat bran, can similarly remain intact in the digestive system like a seed coat or peel. The only difference between hard bran and the seed coat is its ability to absorb water. As it absorbs water it swells and increases stool bulk in the large intestine. Sometimes the fiber can irritate the bowel similar to peels.

Soluble Versus Insoluble Fiber

Does something dissolve in water? That's the first question a student asks of any substance. With dietary fiber it's the most basic means of identifying the two extremes I mentioned: cellulose is insoluble and mucilage is soluble. Other types of fiber fall somewhere in-between. If you dissolve some salt in a glass of water you get a clear solution that looks like pure water. Soluble fiber, in contrast, doesn't always form a "clear" solution, but since it dissolves to some extent, we still say it's "soluble."

In plants, *cellulose* is the basic structure of the cell walls. It protects the inside of the plant cell and provides rigid structure; thus, cellulose is found in just about every plant cell. Cellulose exists wherever structure and strength are required, so it's found in the peels of fruit, such as apples, pears and plums, potato skins, and the matrix and coating of some grains, such as wheat, corn, and seeds (e.g., apple seeds). It's the material this paper is made from; in fact, humans use cellulose mainly to make paper.

Lignins are insoluble and with cellulose they help to impart structure to plants. Wherever there's cellulose in food, there's usually some lignin. Similar to cellulose, we find lignin in grains and potato skins; however, there's no need for it in fruit peels, so fruit contains very little lignin.

Hemicelluloses are in the middle between soluble and

insoluble fiber. ("Hemi" means half.) Hemicelluloses are found with the celluloses. They help to hold the cellulose together and serve as a type of cement. You find them wherever you get cellulose; that's from wheat, whole grains, seeds, and skins.

Pectins, the glue that helps to hold plant cells together and bind water, are soluble. These two functions tell you to look at plant cells that need to retain water because of growing conditions. Think of fruits such as apples, bananas, citrus, and even berries. The water-binding capacity of pectin is illustrated in jelly, which is held firm by just a small pinch of pectin.

Gums are found in plant stems and some seeds. In fact, when these high-gum seeds or stems are moistened, they become gelatinous. Think of oatmeal, kidney beans soaked in water, or zucchini squash; they all exude some gummy type of material. Gums can dissolve almost completely in water. They have excellent water-binding abilities and in fact are used as binders in commercial foods, such as ice creams.

Mucilage gets us to the other extreme of fiber; it's totally soluble. It's found in plant seeds and aquatic plant leaves. Psyllium seed is grown commercially for this type of dietary fiber and is used in fiber supplements, such as Metamucil.

I've summarized this in Table 14.1 which lists the six types of dietary fiber and the common sources of each.

TABLE 14.1
The Six Types of Fiber

Fiber Type	Plant Function	Food Sources
Cellulose (insoluble)	Structure of cell walls	Wheat bran, fruit peels, seed coats
Lignins (insoluble)	Structure of cell walls with cellulose	Cereal grains, potato skins
Hemicellulose (partly soluble)	Holds cells together with cellulose	Wheat bran, grains
Pectins (soluble)	Bind cells together and water	Fruits
Gums (soluble)	Binding substances in stems, seeds, and vegetables	Oatmeal, legumes, vegetables
Mucilages (soluble)	Similar to gums in seeds, aquatic plants	Seaweed, seeds

How Fiber Works for You

Fiber accomplishes four functions that are important to intestinal health: bulking of stools; decreasing flowability of the contents; fermentation by bacteria; adsorption. Adsorption helps fiber remove unwanted dietary materials and substances produced by the body. It's worthwhile to consider each of these functions separately.

Bulking of Stools

All fiber binds water for two reasons: fiber attracts water because of its chemical structure, such as the pectins, and fibers also hold water in their open spaces, like the cellulose fibers of papers. Fiber is seen in the water it binds, and the extent to which it swells up. Most experts believe these properties account for the bulking effect that fiber has on stools.

Because different fiber has different water-binding abilities, it follows that some will bulk stools more than others. For example, wheat-bran cellulose will bulk up to about seven times its size, whereas mucilage from seaweed will bulk up to about 30 times its size. As you can see, mucilage has more than four times the bulking capacity of cellulose.

It's easy to see why a low-fiber diet produces small, hard stools in normal folks. These hard stools contain little water and are simply undigested food and some bacteria from the large intestine. And you can see why the right kind of fiber can produce more consistent stools for folks with chronic diarrhea by binding the water and other components, such as bile acids. You can also understand how the saying "an apple a day" originated, since apples add pectin, a high-bulking fiber, to the diet.

Stool Transit Time

Fibers work both ways on flowability. They speed things up when they're sluggish and slow them down when they're runny. You're probably ahead of me and know it's because of the water-binding capacity. Fiber forms what chemists call a gel. Mucilage gums and pectins do this better than cellulose and hemicelluloses, which barely do it at all.

All fiber will bulk and increase the rate of transit for slow, hard stools by bulking up the stool and adding nature's lubricant, water. Increasing dietary fiber by 10 or 20 percent will produce these effects. The average North American gets about 13 to 15 grams of fiber daily. A large apple a day adds over 3 grams, a 23 percent increase. Because an apple contains almost a gram of soluble fiber and 2 grams of insoluble fiber, it'll increase the bulk of the stool more than 23 percent.

Suppose your problem is the opposite—chronic diarrhea. Fiber can work miracles, but you've got to be selective. The best binding capacity is obtained from the soluble fibers. That means if you ate a bowl of oatmeal you'd add 3 grams of dietary fiber, about two of which are soluble gums. (Not surprisingly, many people with the chronic diarrhea of IBD tell me they feel better when they eat oatmeal.) Better still, you can take a tablespoon of a soluble fiber supplement such as Metamucil and add about 6 grams of soluble fiber immediately. The application of dietary fiber to the chronic diarrhea and watery stools of IBD is the subject of Chapter Five.

Science also explains why old wives' tales advise giving apples and bananas to children when they have diarrhea. The apples add pectin, the bananas add gums, and together they bind up the water and help things slow down. Binding is also accomplished by the use of specialized clay, which does the same thing as soluble dietary fiber. This is not used as frequently as it was in the past.

Another way to slow stools down is to take a fiber supplement that consists of mucilage. There are a number of these supplements on the market made from psyllium seeds. Still another technique used clinically and more frequently at home is the use of plant gums; available either as guar or xantham gums, they bind many times their weight in water and help to stop watery stools. Gums bind better than any other form of fiber and should be used in small amounts with water. The most common, guar gum, is very effective.

Fermentation

Remember the saying: "Beans, beans, the musical fruit, the more you eat the more you toot"? It describes one property of soluble fiber: its ability to be fermented by the bacteria of the large intestine. Beans happen to contain soluble fiber and other materials that are fermented in the large intestine a little better than any other foods. The by-products of the fermentation are gases, such as carbon dioxide, some foul-smelling fatty acids, and water. All these by-products, together with unfermented fiber, are important, and add up to good stools of bulky consistency, that are soft and easily moved. Unfortunately, fermentation produces gas that imparts a bloated feeling. Since all gas passes, it can irritate one's sensibilities, so some soluble fiber has some ascetically unappealing, but not health-detracting qualities.

Taking in the correct amount of dietary fiber and balancing the ratio of soluble fiber to insoluble fiber will produce benefits, bulking stools, slowing down chronic diarrhea, and speeding up chronic constipation. The proper amount of fermentation will add more bulk in the large intestine and help move things along without too much gas.

Adsorption: Getting Rid of Unwanted Materials

Fiber lowers blood cholesterol levels by binding bile acids and dietary cholesterol. Soluble fibers, such as pectins, gums, and mucilage, do it very well; but insoluble fibers, such as cellulose, don't. Fiber also removes certain materials from the digestive tract.

Our liver makes bile acids from cholesterol and passes them into the small intestine to help digest fat. If bile acids don't bind with fiber, they are reabsorbed further down the intestinal tract. This sort of bile-acid recycling stops cholesterol from being converted to bile acids, which means that extra cholesterol is then released into the blood and elevates the blood cholesterol level. By binding the bile acids with dietary fiber, cholesterol is passed in the stools which helps to lower blood cholesterol levels. The fiber also binds dietary cholesterol and passes it out in the stools, which is the main reason we're urged to eat a high-fiber diet for healthy hearts.

During the 1960s, Dr. Ben Ershoff took this theory into the lab at the University of Southern California. He fed rats three different diets. The first group got the control diet—standard rat chow. The second group got a series of toxic diets that contained standard chow mixed with toxic chemicals, such as food dyes and artificial sweeteners. The third group got a series of diets with the chow, the toxic chemicals, and one of several types of fiber.

Rats on the first diet grew well. They thrived and looked normal and fit. Rats on the second group of diets were in very poor shape; only about 15 percent survived and then just barely. They didn't grow, didn't look good, and even the most experienced lab workers felt sorry for them! Rats on the third group of diets did well. Those fed alfalfa fiber did as well as the controls on the first diet. Those that had cellulose did better than those in group two, but not as well as those on either alfalfa or the control diet. As we can see, fiber can bind, and in this case, detoxify chemicals. Alfalfa is a plant that contains a large proportion of soluble fiber (Chapter Twenty-Four). Soluble fiber worked best; insoluble worked least. This study was expanded to many types of fiber.

Dr. Ershoff, in this landmark experiment, proved that dietary fiber could bind toxic chemicals and make a toxic rat diet safe. I'm not suggesting that if you eat harmful things you can add a little fiber and be safe, but fiber, mostly soluble fiber, can bind more than water, bile acids, and cholesterol. It can actually bind toxic materials and render them neutral. It can bind irritants and help remove them from the system with as little difficulty as possible.

Since Dr. Ershoff's experiment, much has been learned. The fiber that binds chemicals best is the soluble, fermentable fiber—pectins, gums, mucilage, and probably some of the hemicelluloses. So, a diet with the correct fiber helps maintain regularity and will help to prevent irritation or even illness.

Effects of Fiber on the Digestive Tract

Feeling Full

What do a large apple and a square of chocolate have in common? Calories! However, you can swallow a square of chocolate in an instant, whereas it takes at least a few minutes even for a teenager to eat the apple. Besides, after you swallow the chocolate, you might want more; after eating the apple, you feel full, satiated. Therefore, the first effect of a high-fiber diet is satiety, satisfying hunger. Fiber-rich foods stay in the stomach longer. We say eating a fiber-rich diet prolongs stomach-emptying time. Soluble fiber seems to do this best. Studies have shown that people feel full longer after a meal rich in soluble fiber as compared to one without fiber or with more cellulose-type fiber. But both types of fiber impart a feeling of fullness.

Chewing high-fiber foods also helps people feel satisfied. The act of chewing seems to satisfy a need that's hard to describe. For example, when people are placed on a complete liquid diet, they miss chewing food within a few days. At the end of a week or more, it's not uncommon for them to ask for an apple.

When you eat food, some digestion begins in the mouth, but accelerates in the stomach. In the stomach, two things happen. The food is thoroughly mixed to a sort of grayish mass called chyme, as acid, enzymes, and mucus produced by the stomach lining are added. Once the contents are thoroughly mixed and enough acid has been produced, the stomach starts emptying its contents into the small intestine. The time between eating and when the food enters the small intestine is called the time of stomach emptying. Fiber slows this process down.

Scientists believe that prolonged satiety is more than simply the delay in stomach emptying, that it's also from bulking in the small intestine. That means that the water and other materials bound to fiber in the stomach pass into the small intestine in the same bulky condition and impart a feeling of fullness. If they do, it explains why the more bulky soluble fiber imparts more satiety.

Transit Time

Transit time is the time between when food first enters your mouth to when its residue appears in the stool. In other words, it's the time from one end to the other! We can break it down further into three phases: the time it spends in the stomach (gastric emptying), the time spent in the small intestine, and the time spent in the large intestine. But to start with a general overview, let's consider total transit time first.

From One End to the Other

Normal adults getting from 35 to 45 grams of fiber each day have an average transit time of about 36 to 48 hours. Let me qualify that. If I made sure that folks got about 40 grams of dietary fiber daily and ate an indigestible marker, say the size of a rice grain, it would appear somewhere between 36 to 48 hours later. In a few people, however, it would show up in 24 hours and in a very few people it would take more than 48 hours. These same people would produce from 150 to 300 grams of stool daily. They might easily have one or two bowel movements daily; after all, 300 grams of stools is two-thirds of a pound and 150 grams is one-third of a pound. That's a fairly large amount.

Variation in Transit Time

Transit time varies in every person and from one person to another. It's different between men and women; in one study where people where monitored, regardless of diet, the average time in women was 25 percent slower than in men. Transit time can vary by two to three times in the same individual or from one group to another, but also can vary from one day to the next for each individual. Stool passage varies widely and there's a large range to what's normal.

Mouth to Large Intestine

Research on the time necessary for food to go from the mouth through the small intestine also proves that people vary widely. But the research studies are consistent, so it gives us insight into what's normal. It seems to take food from 90 to 180 minutes to go from the mouth to its first appearance in the large intestine. That means that when we eat a meal, some of its components might be entering the large intestine in as little as 1½ hours, or possibly a little less. It could also take as much as 3 hours.

Another experiment illustrated the influence of fiber. Adding guar gum to food increased the transit time by 75 minutes, pectin by 15 minutes, and cellulose had no effect. This tells us that the largest amount of time that food spends in our body is its residence in the large intestine. But it also tells us that passage through the small intestine is influenced by fiber—and, to some extent, the pectins—that cause things to gel.

Large Intestine

Let's say that mouth to anus time is 2 days and time from mouth to large intestine is 3 hours. It follows that digested food normally spends about 45 hours or almost 2 days, in the large intestine. Therefore, we should examine what we know about the effect of fiber on the large intestine.

Soluble fiber is more likely to be fermented by the bacteria that reside in the large intestine. Fiber that doesn't get fermented will influence the water content and transit time in the large intestine. The by-products of fermentation will influence the composition of the stool. On a fiber-rich diet, the stool will contain more water, some fatty acids, and gas.

Insoluble fiber—wheat bran for example—decreases transit time through the large intestine. It increases the volume of the stools and makes them easier to pass. By comparison, some soluble fiber doesn't get completely fermented and helps to decrease the transit time. This probably includes the hemicelluloses and some gums, but not pectin.

Intraintestinal Pressure

When stools contain enough fiber, the stool volume is large and the internal pressure is low. People who have small, compact, dry, hard stools have much higher internal pressure than people whose stools are large, soft, and moist. If fermentation produces gas, the pressure is lower when there's sufficient fiber.

Are you wondering why I am telling you this? Intestinal discomfort is always worse when there's additional pressure; normal waves of intestinal motion alone produce pressure. The intestine pushes the stools along. If it's working on small, hard, dry stools, more pressure is generated than if it's working on large, soft, moist stools. If there are any flaws in the lining of the intestine, such as is the case with colitis, ulcerative colitis, or diverticulosis, they are made worse and more painful by high pressure. Conversely, if stools are kept large, soft, and moist, the pressure is lower, the pain is less, and the illness is not made worse. In fact, it's usually relieved.

What's the Take-Away?

Though we'll talk more about applying what we've discussed, this is a good time to visualize what we've learned. Fiber is clearly the critical nutrient of the digestive tract. Although there are other important points to consider, such as cancer prevention, transit time, and producing good stools, relieving diarrhea and constipation are important.

Variety

Both soluble and insoluble fiber are necessary: soluble fiber slows things down from the stomach through the small intestine, whereas insoluble fiber seems to have its greatest influence in the large intestine. Soluble fiber, the great normalizer, seems to slow down in the large intestine passage when it's too fast, but some insoluble fiber is also necessary.

As food, that means lots of pectin gum and mucilage for

the small intestine, and some hemicellulose and cellulose for the large intestine. It's a tall order, but feasible if you take time for careful food selection. For example, oatmeal is a better breakfast cereal than wheat bran, and an apple is a better dessert than cake. Each meal should contain a variety of vegetables, with beans being given a fair chance. This all adds up to the wide variety of vegetable foods. I've summarized the fiber content of some commonly used foods in Table 14.2.

TABLE 14.2
Food Sources of Fiber
Fiber Content Per Serving in Grams

Food	Serving	Soluble	Insoluble	Total
Vegetables:				
Asparagus	¾ c.	0.8	2.3	3.1
Beans:	½ c.			
Green		0.5	1.6	2.1
Kidney		2.5	3.3	5.8
Lima		1.2	3.2	4.4
Pinto		2.0	3.3	5.3
White		1.4	3.6	5.0
Broccoli	½ c.	0.9	1.1	2.0
Brussels sprouts		1.6	2.3	3.9
Cabbage	½ c.	0.9	1.1	2.0
Carrots	½ c.	1.1	1.2	2.3
Cauliflower	½ c.	0.5	1.1	1.6
Celery (raw)	½ c.	0.4	0.9	1.3
Corn (kernels)	½ c.	1.7	2.2	3.9
Eggplant	½ c.	0.8	1.2	2.0
Kale	½ c.	1.4	1.4	2.8
Lettuce (raw)	½ c.	0.1	0.2	0.3
Onions (raw)	½ c.	0.8	1.8	2.6
Peas	½ c.	1.1	3.0	4.1
Potatoes baked:				
Sweet	½ c.	0.7	1.0	1.7

Food	Serving	Soluble	Insoluble	Total
White	½ c.	0.9	0.9	1.8
Radishes	5 med.	0.1	0.5	0.6
Squash:	½ c.			
Acorn		0.5	3.8	4.3
Zucchini		1.3	1.4	2.7
Tomato (raw)	1 med.	0.2	0.6	0.8
Turnip	½ c.	0.8	0.9	1.7
Fruits (raw) with skins:				
Apple	1	0.8	2.0	2.8
Apricots	2	0.7	0.8	1.5
Banana	½ med.	0.3	0.7	1.0
Blackberries	½ c.	0.7	3.8	4.5
Cherries	10	0.3	0.9	1.2
Grapefruit	½ med.	0.6	1.1	1.7
Grapes	12	0.1	0.4	0.5
Orange	1 small	0.3	0.9	1.2
Peach	1 med.	0.6	1.0	1.6
Pear	½ med.	0.5	2.0	2.5
Pineapple	½ c.	0.3	0.9	1.2
Plums	3 small	0.7	1.1	1.8
Raspberries	¾ c.	0.4	6.4	6.8
Strawberries	¾ c.	0.7	1.3	2.0
Grain Products:				
Bread:	1 slice			
French		0.3	0.7	1.0
Rye		0.3	0.6	0.9
White		0.2	0.3	0.5
Whole wheat		0.3	1.1	1.4
Cereal:				
All-Bran	⅓ c.	1.7	6.9	8.6
Shredded wheat	1 square	0.4	2.4	2.8
Oatmeal	⅓ c.	2.0	1.0	3.0
Rice:				
Brown	½ c.	0.2	2.2	2.4
White	½ c.	—	0.1	0.1
Spaghetti	½ c.	0.3	0.5	0.8
Almonds	1 Tbsp.	0.1	1.0	1.1

Putting the Information to Work

A consensus of medical opinion recommends 25 to 45 grams of fiber each day, roughly 30 grams of fiber for a 125-pound person and 40 grams for a 175-pound person. Let's see how that would work out. I've left out all meats and nonvegetable foods and lumped breads together. Table 14.2 shows that it can be done. More important, because vegetables are so modest in Calories, the serving sizes can easily be doubled. Doubling the servings of vegetables and fruit will improve the fiber dramatically.

You might look at my daily fiber menu (Table 14.3) and say, "No way." If you do, you're typical, since the average person gets about 13 to 15 grams of fiber daily—in total. But before you reject the idea, look over what you would have accomplished.

TABLE 14.3
Daily Fiber Menu:
A Plan That Provides Over 35 Grams
of Fiber Without the Use of High-Fiber Cereals

Food	Soluble Fiber	Insoluble Fiber	Total Fiber
Breakfast			
Oatmeal	2.0	1.0	3.0
Grapefruit	0.6	1.1	1.7
Snack			
Banana (1 whole)	0.6	1.4	2.0
Lunch			
Lima beans	1.2	3.2	4.4
Broccoli	1.6	2.3	3.9
Peach	0.6	1.0	1.6
Snack			
Apple	0.8	2.0	2.8

Food	Soluble Fiber	Insoluble Fiber	Total Fiber
Dinner			
Potato	0.7	1.0	1.7
Brussels sprouts	1.6	2.3	3.9
Salad	1.6	2.2	3.8
Melon	0.4	0.6	1.0
Snack			
Pear	0.5	2.0	2.5
Miscellaneous			
Wheat bread (4 slices)	1.2	4.4	5.6
Daily Total			
Total	13.4	24.5	37.9

You'd have achieved an outstanding total of more than 37 grams of fiber and more than 30 percent of it as soluble fiber. With the emphasis on fruit, you'd be likely to get lots of hemicellulose. All that adds up to good intestinal function. In the next chapter we'll look more closely into the use of fiber supplements and some of the negative things to consider.

These data are estimated from various sources. There is still much debate about methods of measuring dietary fiber and the difference between soluble and insoluble fibers. Don't be concerned if these numbers differ from others you have seen; the values are not precise.

CHAPTER FIFTEEN

Water

Water is the most important of all nutrients. We can survive a deficiency of most nutrients for months, but we can last without water for only a few days. It's the only nutrient we also use for recreation and washing. Infants are almost 90 percent water and adults are about 60 percent. If you weigh 120 pounds, you're 72 pounds of water, so when someone says "you're all wet," they're right.

What Water Does for Us

Water expands when it freezes, making ice float. If ice didn't float, life in the water wouldn't survive freezing. Without this unique property of water, life on earth would be quite different. It also means that living human tissue can't be easily frozen.

Water is the major part of our blood; it carries nutrients to each cell and takes materials away. It's part of the structure in each of our body's 50 trillion cells. Each cell is bathed in water, along with a balance of electrolytes.

Water takes part in most body processes. It dissolves protein, amino acids, carbohydrate, and minerals; and there's even a system to get fat into water. For example, before we can use sugar, it enters into a chemical reaction with water in the stomach; much the same is true for the metabolism of fat, protein and other carbohydrates. When we convert chemical energy from food into physical energy, water is produced; we share this property of conversion with automobile engines.

Water's ability to hold heat is important. It helps to keep our body temperature at 98.6°F. When water changes from liquid to gas and evaporates, it absorbs heat. Our natural air-conditioning system of sweat glands helps cool us down. And when we get cold, this system closes up to conserve water and heat.

Hard Versus Soft Water

Tap water can be a good source of minerals. "Hard" water contains calcium, magnesium, and other trace minerals. "Soft" water is usually made by replacing calcium with sodium in most home-softening systems. Excess sodium from water softeners can contribute to high blood pressure in some people and force them to use bottled water in a low-sodium diet. Alternatively, tap water can be made soft by the more expensive methods of distillation and reverse osmosis. These methods, also available for homes, remove all the minerals, including sodium. People living in hard-water areas have a slightly longer life expectancy, probably from the extra calcium, magnesium, and some trace minerals they get in the water. Small amounts of these minerals add up over a lifetime.

Dehydration: Illness

An elaborate system of electrolytes keeps the correct ratio of water inside each cell to the water outside each cell, and the proper amount of water in our blood vessels. The system often becomes unbalanced during illness, especially with the vomiting or diarrhea that usually accompanies flu or food poisoning. Vomiting or diarrhea brings on severe water loss, or dehydration.

Dehydration can be disastrous. When it results from diarrhea or vomiting, essential minerals, especially potassium, are lost with the water and the mineral balance is upset. In severe cases, serious problems develop. And if water is restored too quickly without the correct minerals, water intoxication follows. Although it's different from alcohol intoxication, it appears the same to the casual observer. The only treatment for illness-induced dehydration is to replenish water, potassium, and other minerals.

Chicken Soup to the Rescue

Reversing dehydration is a job for chicken soup. Chicken soup first appeared in China as a remedy for dehydration from flu and digestive upset. When made from the bones and carcass of the chicken, it's an excellent source of water, potassium, magnesium, and some aromatic materials that reduce congestion. It's a universal folk remedy that has been researched. It works! Alas, modern canned and packaged soups don't have the same qualities as homemade chicken soup. With their excess sodium and lack of the other materials, they can even make the problem worse.

Water Loss = Fatigue

Water loss from perspiration can be dangerous for active people, especially dancers. After a workout, body weight often drops by 5 percent. With such a serious water loss, muscular capacity declines 20 to 30 percent, leading to fatigue and a loss of mental alertness. That's why people exercising on a hot day claim their legs get rubbery and they can't think clearly. When you hear of a young jogger or mountain climber having a stroke, it's usually the result of dehydration. Stroke from dehydration has made many Mt. Everest expeditions fail.

Replacing Water Loss

Water loss from activity or even illness is most effectively replaced by plain water. Using salt tablets is an old practice that research has proved *wrong!* Beverages such as Gatorade contain the minerals in sweat: simple sugar and some soluble starch. Advertising implies that they replace fluid loss better than water. Research supports their use only when you're exercising close to maximum capacity for more than 4 hours and very few people, even athletes, do that.

Research proves that the best way to replace fluid is to drink small quantities of water regularly. About a cup—8 ounces or more—of water every hour will do fine, depending on the heat, and so on. It's better to drink 4 or more ounces every 30 minutes. For prolonged activity in the heat, diluted fruit juice is excellent. Food, especially natural fruits and vegetables, also helps to replace the electrolytes potassium and sodium, but processed foods usually contain excess sodium and insufficient potassium.

Thirst

People can't rely on thirst as their only cue to drink water. The need for water precedes the sensation of thirst by as much as an hour. As an insurance policy, the best thing to do is always drink a little water when you're active or if you have diarrhea. The most common dietary reason for poor performance among athletes is not drinking enough water. And very often it's the reason average folks, like you and me, feel tired.

Water for Average Folks

An average 150-pound adult needs about 2 quarts of water daily—that's 64 ounces (8 large glasses). An active person could easily need 80 ounces, or 10 large glasses, daily. The need depends on activity, temperature, altitude, and the use of foods that increase the need for water.

Caffeine and alcohol add to our bodies' water loss. Protein, sugar, and fiber-rich foods call for more water; protein and carbohydrates need it for metabolism; fiber requires water because stools are about 75 percent water. Since you have more stools on a high-fiber diet, you need more water. Most sugar-containing soft drinks taken to quench thirst actually increase your need for water!

Water for IBD Sufferers

Diarrhea is water loss in living (if not beautiful) color! That's correct. Whenever you've got loose, watery stools and have frequent movements, you're losing water. You can't possibly perform to your best with such continuous water loss. You'd always be in a state of mild dehydration. In addition to making you feel tired, such dehydration is an invitation to kidney stones. I wasn't surprised to hear that some people say drinking water stops diarrhea and even stops an IBD flare-up. Restoring water balance helps to stop potassium loss (see Chapter Twenty-one), and that stops diarrhea. It also helps to flush irritants out of the system.

If you live with watery stools or chronic diarrhea, I suggest you treat yourself as if you were an athlete. That means drinking up to 80 ounces of water daily. It sounds like a lot, and it is a lot, but your water loss through stools could easily be that much or more. In addition, be especially careful of the electrolyte balance mentioned in Chapter Twenty-one. Water loss and electrolyte loss go together like milk and honey.

Kidney stones have been discussed in other chapters, but they really belong in a discussion of water. People with IBD often get kidney stones; it's a side effect of the most commonly used medication. The best defense is to keep lots of water going through the kidneys, and to eat potassium-rich foods to guarantee a good electrolyte balance.

Another comment that's frequently heard from people who use medication is "It makes my urine deep yellow." Well, maybe it does, but deep yellow urine may also be highly concentrated urine. Another way to view it is as a need for more water—more reason to treat yourself like an athlete and strive for the 80 ounces I propose.

Who Drinks All that Water?

How much water do you drink? Most people don't drink much water; they get it from beverages, fruits, vegetables, and other foods instead. Our body uses water to get rid of unwanted chemicals. So if you ingest more chemicals, such as sweeteners, colors, flavors, and so on, with the water you drink, the body's water has to go further. Your kidneys have to work harder to conserve the body's water supply. Water is the only nutrient that's good for us in excess.

Our Water Supply

In this decade we've become more concerned about the purity of municipal water supplies. City water usually contains low levels of chlorinated hydrocarbons, nitrates, and unwanted minerals, such as aluminum. These chemicals in drinking water should concern us. Research on the geographical distribution of Alzheimer's disease shows a correlation with aluminum in drinking water. Some water supplies force people to use bottled water or home purification systems in order to follow a low-sodium diet. Chlorinated hydrocarbons and nitrates increase the risk of cancer. At the levels they're found in water, the chances of these unwanted materials creating health problems are minimal—"less than one in a million," we're told. I answer that statement with this: "Every week someone whose chances were less than one in a million wins the lottery!"

Insist that your local water is kept pure.

CHAPTER SIXTEEN

Fat-Soluble Vitamins

A vitamin is an indispensable, noncaloric organic substance, needed in very small amounts, which performs functions essential to health and life. Without vitamins you get sick.

A 150-pound person requires about 100 milligrams of vitamins daily. One-hundred milligrams isn't much; that quantity would just cover the period at the end of this sentence. But 100 milligrams would contain 11 different vitamins!

If you're deficient in a particular vitamin, you'll get sick. If the vitamin isn't restored in time, you'll die. Ancient literature contains many disease descriptions that we know now are simple vitamin deficiencies, but our understanding of vitamins had to await twentieth-century chemistry with its sensitive, analytical techniques.

Chemists separate vitamins into two groups: water soluble and fat soluble, according to whether they dissolve in oil or water. The body stores fat-soluble vitamins in its fatty tissues, where they can accumulate. In contrast, we don't store the water-soluble vitamins, and thus we need more of them daily even though we're always dealing with very small amounts.

How Much We Need: Back to the RDA

Vitamins, like all nutrients, are expressed in recommended daily dietary allowances, RDA for short. The RDAs get more accurate as our knowledge advances. I've included a listing of the most recent RDAs at the end of the book.

Whenever we talk about the RDA on a food label, we're using the U.S. RDA. The U.S. RDA is an RDA established for labeling; it's an average RDA for adults or children. One purpose is to help people make food choices. Shoppers can decide if a packaged food has the nutrition they're looking for and then compare one product with another. A major purpose of the RDA is to help the consumer learn how to use nutrition in food choice. Whenever I talk about the RDA in the context of nutrition, I'm referring to the RDA established by the Food and Nutrition Board. In contrast, whenever I'm discussing a food product, I'm shifting into the U.S. RDA labeling context even if I don't say so. The differences between the two are minor for our purposes and shouldn't cause concern.

Fat-Soluble Vitamins

Fat-soluble vitamins include vitamins A, D, E, and K. Each one is unique and is important for our health. They are stored in fatty tissues of some organs, such as the liver. These tissues are quite stable; therefore, we have a larger supply of these vitamins than most of the water-soluble vitamins.

Vitamin A

In the middle of the handle of the Big Dipper are two closely associated stars, a bright one called Mizar and a very dim one known as Alcor. Long ago in the age of campfires and oil lamps, when the sky over cities was not yet shrouded in electric haze and smog, the Arabs used Alcor as a test of good eyesight. If someone failed the test, they prescribed vegetables, most likely alfalfa, as a remedy. Some 2,400 years ago Hippocrates was aware of this test of night visual acuity. Like the Arabian physicians before him, he sought to improve the night vision of his patients by supplementing the diet, thus following his maxim, "Let food be thy medicine." Instead of using only vegetables, he prescribed liver—calves' liver for those who could barely see Alcor or could see it only occasionally and beef liver for those who could not see the dim star at all. Although he didn't know what the therapeutic factor was, he realized that more of it was present in the liver of old animals than in young ones, characteristic of all fat-soluble vitamins.

Let's look at vitamin A. In European folklore, the benefits of vitamin A were usually associated with the carrot. The carrot is a member of the parsley family, which includes celery and parsnips. It evolved from the weed called Queen Anne's lace. Long recognized as a medicinal plant, the carrot has for centuries been a staple in soups, stews, sauces, and salads. It contains a substance called beta carotene, which is also found in fruits and vegetables, including leafy vegetables. In plants, beta carotene helps trap light for photosynthesis. It is also the basic material from which we make vitamin A. Beta carotene is converted into vitamin A by our intestinal wall and in the liver. So unlike many other vitamins, vitamin A is an animal product, although its basic material, beta carotene, comes from plants.

Vitamin A and Tissue Development

Vitamin A is necessary for cell differentiation, the process by which each of the body's 50 trillion cells specializes and takes on a particular shape and set of complex functions. An especially important role is played by vitamin A in the smooth-surface tissues of the body, including the skin, the mucous membranes, the mouth, the eyes, the nose, and the entire digestive system. The human body has trillions of cells, most of which are continually being replaced. Each one depends on vitamin A to help it develop into what it's supposed to be, whether a cell in the lining of the intestinal tract or a cell in the eye.

Consider, for example, the skin, which is the body's largest organ and covers the entire surface. A skin cell is formed well below the surface that is visible. As it migrates upward, it typically changes from a round "basal" cell to a flattened "squamous" cell when it reaches the surface. It also specializes, depending upon its location; in the nose, the mouth, the stomach, the large intestine, and the small intestine, it becomes a particular kind of mucous membrane. On the face, chest, or arm it differentiates into external skin. The process of differentiation requires vitamin A, the same vitamin A that is made in the liver from beta carotene.

In the eye, the basal cells differentiate into highly specialized surface cells. In the cornea of the eye, for example, the cells must be completely transparent. If they are clouded, it's as if a camera had a dark filter or even a cap over the lens. Visual impairment or blindness occurs when cells in the eye tissue become keratinized—that is, amorphous, dry, and scaly. If you think of a corn or a callus on a toe and imagine eye tissue becoming like this, you will have an idea of what it would be like to be blinded in this way. In some third-world countries where food is scarce, it's estimated that more than 200,000 children become permanently blind each year because of lack of vitamin A.

Hair and fingernails are composed principally of keratin. But in most other tissue, the growth of keratin is devastating. In the life of the large intestine, the integrity of the walls helps to prevent infections and toxic substances from entering the blood; prolonged severe deficiency of vitamin A leads to keratinization of the delicate tissues and cracking of the walls. Cracking of this type can develop in many parts of the alimentary tract from the lips to the anus. Diarrhea begins and the body becomes less able to process food efficiently. Nutrients fail to be absorbed and infection sets in. As the deficiency progresses, external skin lesions may develop along with cracks, peels, and blisters. Eventually death may result.

Vitamin A and Mucus Production

Sensitive tissues, such as the lungs, intestines, and mouth rely upon the secretion of mucus to protect them and to help them perform their special functions. Mucus is the body's lubricant; it helps keep substance moving throughout the digestive system. When vitamin A is deficient, mucus production may stop, the tissue may crack, and infection can begin. If vitamin A is then provided, the tissue barriers to infection can be restored. For this reason, vitamin A has earned the name "the infection fighter," as though it had some kind of antibiotic property. In fact, however, vitamin A acts not by killing germs but by excluding them from vulnerable tissues.

High Beta Carotene Foods and Cancer

People once ascribed certain deaths to a disease they called "the wasting disease." Today we know it as cancer. A myriad of factors are involved in its development. Vitamin A and beta carotene both play a role.

Think of a person living in a coastal village in Japan, or in a reasonably prosperous part of rural Africa, a person who eats unprocessed vegetables, fruits, and cereals more frequently than Americans, and whose protein consists mainly of fish and poultry rather than steaks or chops. Imagine that this person's brother emigrates to the United States or to western Europe, where the air is heavy with factory fumes, auto exhaust, and cigarette smoke, and where the diet is much higher in fats and sugar at the expense of vegetables. The man residing in the modern world has 10 to 15 times the risk of developing cancer as his brother back home.

Many factors are involved in the development of cancer.

There is no one direct "cause," but the risk of cancer may be increased by not eating fresh fruits and vegetables. In addition to fiber, carrots and other fruits and vegetables provide many dietary factors, among them beta carotene. The standard American diet is generally deficient in beta carotene-rich foods. No one would claim that cancer is caused by the absence of carrots, red cabbage, sweet potatoes, green leafy vegetables, or liver, much less that it can be cured by eating these foods or by taking beta carotene capsules. Consider, however, Dr. Richard Shekelle's studies on heavy smokers. One group followed a diet typical of the United States, whereas the other group had a more vegetarian diet, rich in beta carotene and fiber. Although the second group consuming a diet rich in beta carotene and fiber had a higher rate of cancer than the average population of nonsmokers, this rate was substantially below that of their fellow heavy smokers, who were eating a typical U.S. diet with its fat and sugar. The dietary factor that made the difference was beta carotene.

A nutrient in its own right, beta carotene is found in all the membrane tissues of the body, including the skin, the eyes, the intestines, lungs, and others. It protects these organs from chemical fumes that are found in the industrialized areas or are ingested with our food. Beta carotene has been shown to reduce the risk of certain types of cancer, such as skin, lung, intestinal, and bladder cancer. Thus, science is uncovering an important role for beta carotene.

Not all of beta carotene's functions are so dramatic, but they do make life more pleasant. Beta carotene also reduces the risk of sunburn and cataracts of the eyes. These benefits are derived from its ability to interact with ultraviolet light from the sun.

More About Beta Carotene

Beta carotene is found in fruits and vegetables; it gives carrots, yams, pumpkins, melons, and oranges their color. It is fat-soluble and stored in fatty tissue throughout the body, including the fat stores just under the skin. In fact, if you regularly drank a large amount of fresh carrot juice, certain parts of your skin would turn a slightly orange color. When the body needs vitamin A, it simply converts some of this beta carotene to the vitamin. As long as beta carotene is available, the body can make as much vitamin A as it requires. However, the body does not have a means of excreting excess levels of preformed vitamin A, which are ingested directly in the form of fish-liver oil or animal liver, or in food supplements; thus, although large quantities of vitamin A itself can be toxic, large amounts of beta carotene are completely safe. Indeed, the orange color is not unsafe, it's just a color.

Who Needs Beta Carotene?

In today's world, two broad classes of people are not obtaining sufficient beta carotene and vitamin A foods. One group consists of impoverished people, who are unable to get the right kinds of foods and obtain the necessary nutrients. Severe deficiency in these groups accounts for about 25,000 deaths per year. The other group of people who are affected (although more subtly or indirectly) by this type of dietary inadequacy, are among the richest in the world and live in economically developed countries. A recent survey showed that 30 percent of Americans get insufficient beta carotene or vitamin A, probably because they lack vegetables and seasonal fruits in their diet. We don't eat organ meats anymore, which also accounts for the shortfall in vitamin A. This decline in organ meat is good for other reasons, but people should make up for it by eating more vegetables.

Even if we get enough beta carotene to preserve our night vision and to facilitate cell differentiation in order to meet the government's criteria of satisfactory health, we still may not be digesting sufficient quantities. Given the toxicity of auto exhaust, factory fumes, and power-plant emissions, I believe there is no one living in U.S. cities who doesn't "smoke." It is, of course, wise to avoid smoking and inhaling "second-hand" smoke and other pollutants. To the degree that modern life requires antioxidant protection against these oxidative pollutants and carcinogens, I believe that beta carotene should be considered not simply the basic material for vitamin A production, but as a nutrient in its own right, with important antioxidant properties. In addition to the question of how much vitamin A we need, we should also ask how much beta carotene the body needs, not only to produce vitamin A, but to perform additional antioxidant functions.

Toxicity of Vitamin A: Safety of Beta Carotene

Excessive vitamin A, such as 50,000 I.U. per day taken regularly for months, can cause serious medical problems. Sometimes even lower amounts may cause problems. The greatest danger is to infants and children. An excess of vitamin A can actually cause death. On one polar expedition, members became seriously disabled and some died after eating bear liver. It seems the polar bear eats so much fish and its liver is so large, that it contains enough vitamin A to poison humans. At all ages, excessive vitamin A intake can cause joint pain, rash, itchiness, an enlarged liver, loss of appetite, and, in women, cessation of menstruation. The symptoms disappear very quickly when the vitamin A intake stops. In contrast to vitamin A, an elevated level of beta carotene may produce a slightly orange skin, but it does not produce vitamin A toxicity. About 60,000 I.U. of beta carotene daily are required to get slightly orange skin. That's a lot of beta carotene and requires beta-carotene supplements or large amounts of carrot juice. People have achieved the orange skin color with capsules of beta carotene and even with carrot juice, and every medical indication shows that they are very healthy with absolutely no toxic symptoms.

Vitamin A, Beta Carotene and IBD

I think in terms of beta carotene, but the convention of the RDA says I should speak in Vitamin A terminology. Now I'm speaking to you about the need for beta carotene; take care of that and vitamin A will be taken care of thanks to your liver. I believe that people with IBD need more beta carotene than average; 25,000 International Units daily are sufficient.

These conclusions derive from the following facts: increased risk of intestinal cancer; chronic diarrhea; loss of dietary fat; and the likelihood of higher than normal intestinal cell turnover. In my mind, it adds up to a simple conclusion: the extra beta carotene can't possibly do any harm and it has the potential to help reduce each of the risks.

Twenty-five thousand I.U. of beta carotene means getting the 2,500 to 5,000 I.U. of vitamin A as a supplement described in Chapter Seven. Beyond that, try eating vegetables and fruit (especially those that are orange and yellow) at each meal every day; for example, a slice of melon or a banana at breakfast and some vegetables and fruit at every other meal. If you can't eat sufficient colored vegetables, I recommend a beta-carotene supplement that contains at least 10,000 I.U. per capsule (see Chapter Seven).

Vitamin D: Sun Worship

The streets of thirteenth-century Weistar, East Germany, were so narrow that most windows admitted very little direct sunlight. Weistar streets were just wide enough for a horse-drawn cart and didn't allow the sun to reach the inside windows, except when it was nearly overhead in the summer. During the winter the residents had little access to sunlight except on their faces and hands when they went out of doors. The winter sun in that part of the world is too low in the sky to be of much value, because when the sun is at an oblique angle, ultraviolet light is severely reduced by the atmosphere. Therefore, the end of winter was nearly the only time when people in northern European cities could receive ample sunshine. Sunshine is essential for vitamin D; sun-worship probably has roots in the human body's need for the sunshine vitamin, not in religion, as many people believe.

The women in Weistar had a saying "Every child must get the January sun." In the coldest part of winter, mothers would carry their children to a park and disrobe them as much as possible to expose them to the sun. Adults got enough sun in the course of their daily activities, but over the years, mothers had noticed that babies born in the fall had a lower rate of survival than babies born in the spring, and that among "winter children" who survived, there was a higher rate of deformities. At first people thought the cause might be the cold or the winter diet, but folk wisdom said it was the scarcity of sunlight. Thus, the older women advised the mothers of winter babies to watch for a day without too much wind, when the temperature was warm for the season, and then let those little bodies soak up the sun.

When historians examined the Weistar church records, they found that a child born in the late fall had the lowest chance of survival. Inscriptions on gravestones showed that more children died in the winter than in the spring. Anthropologists who examined the actual bones of the deformed children confirmed *rickets*, the classical vitamin-D-deficiency disease. Having been conceived in April or May was a disadvantage, because it meant being born in the winter months, when the sun was low and people stayed indoors. In contrast, the autumn baby could store enough vitamin D in its liver to get through the winter. The winter baby would be faced with not getting enough vitamin D during the most important growth period and deformities were the result. Since mother's milk didn't have enough vitamin D, the January sun was necessary.

Industrial Society

In nineteenth-century England, during the Industrial Revolution, smoke and high buildings darkened the skies of the cities. Unable to get adequate sunlight, many children developed bow legs and poorly formed arms, hands, and feet. Tiny Tim, the character created by Charles Dickens, was a product of these conditions. During the 1920s and 1930s, while children in Detroit and other northern industrial centers throughout the world were suffering from rickets, the science of nutrition showed the necessity of supplementing the diet with vitamin D.

At first vitamin D was added to bread, but this was not effective. But while nearly all children eat bread, there's another food that every child needs in order to develop strong bones. This, of course, is milk, and it's the best vehicle for vitamin D because absorption of the vitamin is more effective in a substance that contains some fat. Even low-fat milk has enough. By 1935, after vitamin D was added to milk, the incidence of rickets in children declined from over 20 percent to barely detectable levels. Milk fortified with vitamin D ranks among the triumphs of nutritional science.

Rickets has, for all practical purposes, been eliminated in affluent countries through the fortification of milk. The disease would reappear, however, if the fortification of milk was omitted. In the 1950s, Scotland learned this lesson when the government decided that butter alone would be an adequate source of vitamin D, so they stopped fortifying the milk supply. Within a few years the medical profession began reporting an alarming incidence of rickets, and the milk program was restored.

Surprisingly, rickets still persists in England, especially in Moslem immigrants from countries where drinking milk is uncommon. Although the sun in their native countries is so high in the sky that the smallest amount of exposed skin is sufficient for the body to make enough vitamin D, Moslem women who move to England don't expose enough of their skin to get the benefit of sunlight. This low level requires exposure of a larger area of skin than that to which these women are accustomed because of their dress tradition.

O Dem Bones

Bones consist of calcium and phosphorus set in a protein matrix called collagen. The word *collagen* is based upon a root meaning "glue" (a boiled bone literally does yield glue), but collagen should be regarded less as an adhesive that holds calcium and phosphorus together than as a structure within which these rigid bone materials are found.

Vitamin D is essential for calcium absorption. When sunlight strikes the skin, the vitamin is activated, then converted into a material that transports calcium across the intestine into the bloodstream. Along with calcium, this material helps the body absorb phosphorus. Vitamin D also works with other hormones to help regulate calcium distribution in the body.

This entire process is necessary, not only to growing children, but also adults. Throughout life cells are constantly being replaced and calcium is being released into the blood and flushed out of the body. Calcium needs to be replaced throughout the life span, and this can happen only with the help of vitamin D. If we are deficient in vitamin D, we cannot absorb enough calcium even if dietary sources are adequate. The result in adults is *osteomalacia*, or soft bones (not to be confused with osteoporosis, a condition caused not only by a lack of vitamin D, but by other factors, including a lack of calcium in the diet).

Osteomalacia occurs most frequently among women from less-developed countries during pregnancy and lactation. If a woman stays indoors, becomes deficient in vitamin D, and thus can't absorb dietary calcium, her body borrows the mineral from her bones. The alveolar bone, the lower jawbone that supports the teeth, is one of the first tissues to give up its calcium. Teeth loosen and the gums become infected, resulting in loss of teeth. Human vertebrae in the back also have a spongy matrix somewhat similar to, although not the same as, the alveolar bone. When calcium or vitamin D is deficient, the vertebrate also gives up calcium. Low back pain can result from lifelong dietary calcium inadequacies and numerous pregnancies.

Further, a level of vitamin D sufficient to sustain a woman prior to pregnancy may be too low when she is carrying a baby. The offspring benefits at the expense of the parent: if the mother does not absorb sufficient dietary calcium to provide for the baby's needs, either while it's in the womb or while she's breast feeding, her body will begin reabsorbing calcium from its own bones and supplying it to the child. If this happens, the mother needs a good supply of vitamin D and calcium to replace what has been lost; otherwise, she can suffer permanent bone damage.

Children are especially vulnerable to a vitamin-D deficiency because their bones are developing fast—an infant doubles its size in the first year, whereas adult bones only need to maintain their integrity. Because bone growth involves proper mineralization of bone, one outgrowth of vitamin-D deficiency, such as rickets in children, is bow legs. Similarly, the ribs may fail to develop adequately, and even the skull can be malformed. At its worst, this disease can result in death; at a more subtle level, rickets can be restricted to poor joint formation, which can be detected only through extensive X-ray analysis by an orthopedic physician.

Although rickets was first identified in 1650, very little was known about the disease until the late nineteenth century, when scientists studied the bones of children who had died from the disease. Between about 1890 and 1920, researchers began to rediscover what the women of Weistar had somehow known: rickets could be avoided by exposure to sunlight. They also found that even artificial light could help, if it was rich in the ultraviolet rays. It was not until 1922 that scientists proved that the anti-ricket effect of cod-liver oil was not dependent upon vitamin A, as it was thought, but upon some other factor. That other factor turned out to be vitamin D.

Excess Vitamin D and Toxicity

Although we have been focusing on vitamin-D deficiency, excessive amounts can cause problems as well, as in the case of vitamin A. It is important to stay within the RDA of 400 International Units of vitamin D per day. If a person consumes more than 2,000 units—five times the recommended level—over a long period of time, the body absorbs correspondingly excessive amounts of calcium, which have to be excreted, placing a strain upon the kidneys. If the strain is severe, the kidneys can fail; and kidney failure can cause death.

Vitamin-D toxicity symptoms include diarrhea, headache, and nausea; if overdose continues to occur, calcium deposits form in the soft tissues of the body as the vitamin mobilizes too much mineral from the bone. Obviously, this can occur most easily in infants, whose overzealous mothers may believe that if something is good, a little more is better. Vitamin-D toxicity is dangerous, because it's rarely observed and physicians may overlook it as they seek other causes for the vague symptoms that I've described. Thus, vitamin-D toxicity should be carefully avoided.

Vitamin D in the Present

As the twentieth century enters its twilight years, vitamin D is taken for granted. In some places the main source is the sun, but for at least part of the year we rely mainly upon the vitamin D added to milk or provided through supplementation. Think about why this is so. A person can live in a Chicago apartment, travel to New York for a meeting, go out for dinner and return home, all without ever going out into the sunlight. Hotels have covered atriums or interior lobbies; airports have underground parking and covered areas where taxis pick up and discharge passengers. Schoolchildren spend most of their day in the classroom, are often driven to and from school in automobiles or buses, and are involved in indoor activities in late afternoon. Even their exercise is often taken inside a large gymnasium. If TV sets could activate vitamin D, most of us would never have to worry about our supply, but during the 4 to 8 hours that many people watch TV, they seldom do so in the sun.

Many people are true "sun worshipers" during the summer months, and among those who can afford the luxury of a trip to the Caribbean or Hawaii, during the winter months as well. Recently we have been warned about the risk of skin cancer from excessive exposure to ultraviolet light. Instead of settling for moderate exposure, some people now go to the other extreme and avoid the sun as much as possible.

It would be nice if we could provide measured and convenient indoor sources of ultraviolet light, especially for people who are institutionalized, who work in offices, or who stay indoors all day. I could even imagine a law that would require that a certain quota of artificial sunlight be made available to office workers or schoolchildren under all conditions. However, this would involve yet another set of regulations. It would be more expensive than a vitamin-D supplement and it would not necessarily create an automatic link with the ingestion of calcium.

So we come back to the question of dietary sources. Like vitamin A, vitamin D is an animal product, but it cannot be made by the body from a vegetable source in the same way that vitamin A can be created by beta carotene. Vitamin D is found in dairy products, such as milk, cream, butter, and eggs, and in organ meats, such as liver and kidney. Oily fish is an especially rich source. In northern Europe the need for vitamin D was the underlying nutritional reason for the Catholic practice of eating fish every Friday.

Is Vitamin D Really a Hormone?

The strange thing about vitamin D is that, since the human body can make its own supply, it may not qualify as a vitamin at all. Apart from dietary cholesterol, the liver makes all the cholesterol the body needs; some of it is carried by the blood to the skin, where, struck by the ultraviolet rays of the sunlight, it is converted to vitamin D. The vitamin is then further converted by the kidneys and the liver into active forms that help the body to absorb calcium and deposit it in the appropriate areas. In this process both the cholesterol and vitamin D are made by the body itself. All that's required from the outside is sunlight. That's why vitamin D is regarded as the sunshine vitamin. Only when we fail to get adequate sunlight do we need to ingest vitamin D.

Vitamin D and IBD

We know that vitamin D and calcium are necessary for good health. People who don't get the RDA of either have increased risk of cancer. People with IBD risk losing dietary vitamin D because they're likely to avoid dairy products, and some will not eat oily fish. Therefore, sunlight and supplements are necessary. In fact, vitamin D could be one reason why people in Sunbelt states have a lower risk of getting intestinal cancer. If you remember that moderate sunlight (especially in winter) is important and follow my supplement plan, you can forget about vitamin D.

Vitamin E: Of Rats and Men

Over the years, nutritional science has changed and rechanged its theories on how vitamin E works. In 1922, vitamin E was identified as a key factor in the fertility of rats; rats deprived of it couldn't reproduce. So when vitamin E was finally isolated in 1936, its association with reproduction led to its being named "tocopherol," meaning in Greek, "to give birth." During the next decade, other dramatic vitamin-E deficiency symptoms were found in animals; these symptoms included heart damage in calves, retarded growth in rabbits, and liver degeneration and muscular dystrophy in chicks and rabbits. There was great hope that similar ailments in humans were also caused by vitamin-E deficiency, so that supplying the vitamin would make the ailments disappear.

No such luck. No vitamin-E deficiency or deficiency diseases were ever found in humans. The government even went so far as to keep volunteers on a low-vitamin-E diet for six years, beginning in 1953. They were watched closely for physical or mental effects. Nothing happened, so E became a vitamin in search of a disease. People afflicted with muscular dystrophy were tested, but it turned out that their tissues contained as much vitamin E as those people without the disease. Therefore, there is no evidence that muscular dystrophy in humans is associated with vitamin-E deficiency.

In 1970, one scientist said, "Vitamin E is one of those embarrassing vitamins that has been identified, isolated, and synthesized by physiologists and biochemists, and then handed to the medical profession with the suggestion that a use should be found for it." All the emotional claims and counterclaims surrounding vitamin E intrigued scientists. They suspected that this vitamin definitely had important uses that they had not as yet discovered. The answers are finally coming into focus.

Vitamin E: What Is It?

Vitamin E is actually a complex of eight substances: four tocopherols and four tocotrienols, thick, light-yellow oils, insoluble in water, resistant to heat, but readily destroyed by such conditions as ultraviolet light, sunlight, freezing, and prolonged exposure to air. The four substances to keep in mind are the tocopherols, named for the first four letters in the Greek alphabet—alpha, beta, gamma, delta. Although the exact effectiveness of the other tocopherols has not been established, it appears that alpha-tocopherol is responsible for 80 percent of vitamin-E activity.

How Vitamin E Works

Unlike most other vitamins, vitamin E does not help break down food or energy. It does not function as a coenzyme in metabolism like vitamins A, C, and the B complex. Vitamin E does become converted to energy when it's taken in large excess.

Oxygen in the body burns food for energy, just as we burn wood for fuel in the fireplace or gasoline for fuel in an engine. In the body, the other vitamins help this process happen. We say that the food is "oxidized." But sometimes oxygen doesn't stop there. Even after a metabolic reaction has taken place, some oxygen molecules continue to break things down. They have no "off" switch. Once fuel is "burned," oxygen molecules generate destructive compounds that attack cells and cell membranes. If unchecked, these "free radicals" can destroy nutrients stored in cells and cause cell damage.

Fats and the essential fatty acids that comprise them are particularly vulnerable to oxidation. This is true not only in the body, but in foods as well. No doubt you've had a bottle of oil or a bag of potato chips that turned rancid. That rancidity is the effect of oxidation on the fatty acids in the vegetable oils.

Vitamin E comes to the rescue. It is a powerful antioxidant, which is why it's found naturally in polyunsaturated oils. It acts as a kind of scavenger for the destructive substances that would otherwise react with the oil and cause decomposition. Scientists recently learned that a trace mineral, selenium, works together with vitamin E in such a way that one enhances the antioxidant activity of the other.

Vitamin E also acts as an antioxidant in the body. For example, vitamin E protects the omega-3 and the omega-6 polyunsaturated oils, discussed in Chapter Twelve, from destruction by oxidation. It protects the polyunsaturated fats in all the cell membranes of the body; otherwise, these fatty components would become "rancid"—that is, undergo oxidation just like other fats and oils. Supplies of vitamin E are distributed throughout the body. Each of our trillions of cells contain some vitamin E in the fatty-cell membranes.

But although it is one of the most effective natural antioxidants in the world, vitamin E is not inexhaustible. If continuously bombarded by enormous amounts of oxygen, it can be overwhelmed and oxidized itself. That's why you need to put the cap back on the bottle of oil, and why it's a good idea to maintain optimum levels of vitamin E in your body.

If you increase the amount of polyunsaturated fats in your diet, you increase your need for vitamin E; in most cases this is easy to do, because they occur in the same foods. But if you eat foods such as frozen french fries or doughnuts, which are high in these fats but have lost their vitamin E, you need to increase your intake of vitamin E-rich foods.

Vitamin E and Premature Infants

Because of its antioxidant function, vitamin E helps doctors save the lives of premature infants, many of whom are anemic. These infants simply haven't had enough time to build iron-rich red blood cells to transport oxygen. At one time doctors tried improving the oxygen intake of premature infants by giving them iron. The infants' bodies were less able to cope with oxidation triggered by the oxygen, however, because they had low levels of vitamin E, which doesn't increase until the third trimester. Without adequate vitamin E, the membranes of the red blood cells were weakened and the cells were destroyed. Adding vitamin E to the iron supplement helped solve the problem. It enabled preterm infants to receive the high concentrations of iron they need to survive, with less risk of oxidation damage.

It was this discovery in 1965 that helped to illuminate vitamin E's antioxidation function. Premature infants were the first humans discovered to be suffering from a lack of this vitamin. In trying to help them, scientists learned some of the ways in which vitamin E sustains human health. Some scientists believe that low levels of vitamin E in premature infant cell membranes can cause eye damage or even blindness when the baby is exposed to a rich oxygen supply. If doctors use supplemental vitamin E, however, this type of oxidation may be preventable. More research is needed in this area.

Vitamin E, Cystic Fibrosis, and Sickle-Cell Disease

Besides premature infants, patients with cystic fibrosis often have great difficulty absorbing vitamin E, which is fat-soluble, as well as other fat and fat-soluble vitamins. Lack of vitamin E's antioxidant protection may mean shortened red-blood cell survival. To extrapolate from red cells to other tissues is a major step. Vitamin E helps protect smokers from getting lung cancer. Smoke contains oxidizing agents that irritate lung cells and the entire lung tissues. Vitamin E reduces the irritation dramatically and helps prevent the cancer. This is an excellent example of vitamin E's protective effects in action.

Vitamin E has also been shown by Dr. Clayton Natta to be in short supply in patients with sickle-cell anemia. Sickle-cell disease predisposes red blood cells to oxidative damage. In this study, 10 out of 13 sickle-cell anemia patients were found to be deficient in vitamin E.

Can Vitamin E Protect Us from Pollution?

Take a deep breath. If you're like most Americans, you live in a bustling metropolitan or suburban area and you've just inhaled air that you might be able to see, air that contains nitrogen oxides, sulfur oxides, and ozone. Once inside your lungs, these chemicals react with fatty acids to generate harmful free radicals. Once this process starts, it becomes a chain reaction. As environmental pollution worsened in the last few decades, many scientists examined vitamin E's antioxidant functions, hoping to find some biochemical armor against pollution. Since the 1970s, increasing numbers of scientists have come to believe that vitamin E's gift to modern health could be its antioxidant protection against air pollution.

Because scientists can't set up experiments to expose human subjects to harmful substances, data on vitamin E and pollution in humans are limited. But studies in numerous laboratories, on several species of animals, show that vitamin E has a definite effect on the survival of those exposed to either ozone or nitrogen dioxide.

Animals with low vitamin-E levels are 3 to 10 times as sensitive to pollution effects as animals given large amounts of vitamin E supplements. This has not been shown to be true of humans. However, in one of the few human studies on vitamin E and pollution, conducted by Dr. A. L. Tappel, 10 subjects were exposed to the pollutant ozone while bicycling in a controlled environment. Large amounts of vitamin E were found to lower the level of oxidation by-products present in the subjects' expired breath. Many of the basic features of these tests are similar enough to conditions affecting urban dwellers to warrant our applying the results to humans. Vitamin E may be among our most important defense systems against oxidant lung injury from the polluted air we breathe.

The Myth of Vitamin E and Sex

How did vitamin E get its undeserved reputation as the sex vitamin? When lack of vitamin E became associated with sterility in male rats and miscarriage in female rats, some people fervently hoped that vitamin E supplements would cure human sterility. Once vitamin E and sex were linked in people's minds, it was only natural to credit vitamin E with improving virility and sexual stamina. Recall, though, that the rats' reproductive problems, leading to the discovery of vitamin E, were the result of total deprivation of this vitamin for an extended time. It is unlikely that any human diet could possibly be deficient enough to lead to such severe problems.

Admittedly, research in this area is complicated. For one thing, it is difficult to conduct the appropriate tests that are needed for scientific proof on humans. Also, much of human sexuality depends on the psychological, so we must take into account the placebo effect. If a person believes something will work, it just may. The placebo effect is so strong that in most bona fide clinical tests on nutrients and medications, scientists arrange to have some subjects given an identical "dummy" pill so that no one, including the experimenter, knows who gets the real thing. Hence, no one's confidence in the treatment will skew the results. So far as we can tell, however, vitamin E has no proven value in preventing sterility or miscarriage in humans.

Vitamin E, Circulation, and Leg Pains

In the mid-1940s, many people believed that vitamin E could cure most heart ailments. Entire clinics devoted to this idea opened. Even though this belief persists today, the scientific evidence behind it is questionable. In a half-dozen studies, patients with chronic chest pains and hypertensive and arteriosclerotic heart disease were given vitamin E and placebos. No positive effects of vitamin E were observed.

However, Dr. K. Haeger and other scientists have found that supplemental vitamin E relieves leg muscle pains, primarily in the calves. This is usually referred to as "claudication pain," most often caused by a narrowing of the arteries in the leg. The question of whether vitamin E has an effect on circulation is unresolved.

Vitamin E and Lung Cancer

By now you're used to the concept of an antioxidant. A little reasoning will lead you to ask: "Does vitamin E reduce the risk of lung cancer?" The answer seems to be "yes!" Vitamin E and the mineral selenium, which we'll discuss in Chapter Twenty, work together to protect lung tissues from toxic fumes, specifically cigarette smoke. Although the evidence is incomplete, the tissues of lung cancer victims who smoked contain less vitamin E and selenium than those of nonsmokers. This, and other findings, strongly suggest that vitamin E, especially with selenium, does help to reduce the risk of lung cancer.

Which Foods Contain Vitamin E?

If we examine nutrition folklore and food customs around the world, we find no folk traditions for obtaining sufficient vitamin E in the diet. Nearly all other vitamins and most minerals have a rich history that has been passed down from generation to generation. This suggests that vitamin E is not difficult to get from food. In fact, vitamin E abounds in the diet. The richest sources include grains, nuts, seeds, and beans, as well as the oils made from them. And whenever you get beta carotene, you also get vitamin E.

Wheat germ oil is the best natural source, providing about 28 I.U. per tablespoon. The recommended dietary allowance (RDA) for adults is 12 to 15 I.U. Whole grains and leafy green vegetables are also good sources. A few oils, such as corn oil, are relatively high in gamma-tocopherol, not alpha-tocopherol, and therefore, are less effective than other oils in contributing active vitamin E to the diet. Consuming a variety of oils and natural foods usually ensures meeting RDA levels.

In a typical American diet, about 65 percent of vitamin E comes from salad oils, shortening, margarine, and other fats and oils. But a refined diet that excludes whole grains and fresh vegetables may not provide the RDA for vitamin E. For example, as much as 80 percent is lost when whole wheat is converted to white bread. Freezing vegetables causes some vitamin-E destruction; deep-fat frying destroys it as well. Even with these cooking, processing, and storing methods, though, the chances are that you'll still get enough vitamin E. Although the symptoms of vitamin-E deficiency have not been identified, conversely, we don't know what benefits it's capable of providing.

IBD and Vitamin E

There have never been any reported effects of vitamin E on IBD and I don't expect any in the next quarter century or so. However, there's a possibility that a person with IBD could fall short of vitamin E. I conclude this from the reduced fat absorption that accompanies the illness. Vitamin E is an oil and is absorbed like all oils and fat. Therefore, sensible supplementation is beneficial.

One problem with a nutrient like vitamin E is the difficulty of knowing what happens when there's not enough. In the early studies researchers didn't know what to look for, but the new evidence suggests that the result could be lung cancer or other forms of cancer. These scientific findings can't be expressed in precise terms yet. Therefore, I suggest trying to get sufficient vitamin E on the basis of the existing evidence. Doubtless more concrete evidence will emerge as science moves forward.

Vitamin K: The Forgettable Vitamin

The need for vitamin K is small—70 to 140 micrograms per day for adults. Our own intestinal bacteria produces much of what we need, and the rest comes from our diet. An average diet, along with this bacterial action, appears to provide 300 to 500 micrograms daily, or at least three times our requirement. A potential problem exists for people who have had large parts of their intestines removed, however; they might not be getting enough vitamin K because the bacteria is missing along with the intestine. The only way to tell for sure is to have a blood test taken. Your doctor is the best judge.

What Does Vitamin K Do?

In 1936, two separate teams of scientists, one in Denmark and one in California, independently discovered vitamin K within a few months of each other. Without this substance, chickens could not form blood clots and developed severe hemorrhage problems. In 1939, vitamin K was isolated in pure form from alfalfa. Because this fat-soluble vitamin proved to be essential to proper coagulation of blood, the Danish scientists decided to call it Vitamin K for *koagulation*, the Danish and German spelling of the word. In healthy individuals, vitamin K works in the liver to form at least six different proteins necessary for blood clotting.

Vitamin K in Foods

If you want further proof that vitamin K is not a problem for most of us, here it is. The foods that are rich in vitamin K include liver and green leafy vegetables, such as spinach, kale, turnip greens, dark green lettuce, and broccoli; and vegetables such as cauliflower and cabbage. Many people do not eat these foods on a daily basis. Also, very little vitamin K is present in most cereals, fruits, carrots, peas, peanuts, oils, most meats, and highly refined foods. Yet there are no vitamin K deficiencies in a normal, healthy population.

IBD and Vitamin K

People who have difficulty absorbing fats may need vitamin K supplements, and people who have had much of their colon or large intestine removed could have a special need for vitamin K. You already know the reason: the intestinal bacteria makes about 50 percent of our vitamin K. Therefore, if there's no large intestine, there's no vitamin K. If a need exists for supplemental vitamin K, your doctor can write a prescription for you. Be sure to ask about this in your discussions.

Antibiotics destroy good bacteria along with bad bacteria, so prolonged use of any antibiotics can pose a vitamin-K problem by killing bacteria. People with IBD must frequently take antibiotics and may need to take supplemental vitamin K. Once again, if the subject of vitamin K doesn't come up, then be sure to ask!

CHAPTER SEVENTEEN

Water-Soluble Vitamins

Vitamin C and eight members of the B complex of vitamins are the water-soluble vitamins. Unlike the fat-soluble vitamins, they are not stored in the body. You need them every day.

Vitamin C: From Limeys to Linus

We associate scurvy, characterized by lethargy, swollen joints, bleeding gums, skin ulcers, and finally death, with vitamin C-deficiency. Actually, these symptoms are what a scientist today would call "moribund symptoms"—the symptoms that appear when a person is near death. The early symptoms are fatigue, lethargy, and susceptibility to colds and other infections.

During the age of seafaring, when Spain and England competed on the high seas, more sailors were lost to scurvy than to battles or typhoons. For example, when the Portuguese explorer Vasco da Gama made his famed voyage around the Cape of Good Hope at the end of the fifteenth century, nearly two-thirds of his crew perished from scurvy. At the same time, the Italian explorer Amerigo Vespucci was on his way to the Americas. Instead of keeping sick crew aboard and letting them die, he put them ashore on an island inhabited by friendly natives, who gave the sailors fresh fruit. Months later, Vespucci returned to the island and found the sailors healthy; their recovery was thought to be so miraculous that he named the island Curaçao, which means "cure." This name was then used by the Indians, the Arawaks, who inhabited the island.

Scurvy is one of humanity's oldest diseases. Accounts of this disease date back to 1500 B.C. Aristotle described it in great detail around 350 B.C., noting such symptoms as lack of energy, inflamed and bleeding gums, and tooth loss. With impeccable Aristotelian logic, the great philosopher reasoned that if figs brought about tooth decay as he had discovered, then something else in the diet must cause loosened teeth and bleeding gums. He did not realize that this slow, painful illness was the result of something *missing* from the diet.

Rose Hips, Bark Tea, Raw Fish

For centuries, central and southern Europeans suffered from vitamin C-deficiency due to a sparse supply of fresh fruits and vegetables. In contrast, other cultures developed ways to supplement their diets with enough vitamin C to avoid scurvy. In some of the cold northern regions of the ancient world, such as China, Mongolia, Siberia, and Scandinavia, people harvested rose hips—the fruits of the wild rose, a flower that grows abundantly in cool climates. They would dry these fruits, grind them into a powder, then make the powder into tea or soup and add it to other foods throughout the long winter months. This custom helped the Swedes when citrus fruits from Italy and Spain were cut off during World War II. *Nypon Sopa*, or rose hip soup, was their primary source of vitamin C until the war ended and trade resumed.

Other plants also yield a supply of the anti-scurvy vitamin. In the West Indies, for example, people relied on a kind of cherry called acerola, and in the evergreen forests of North America, natives brewed a vitamin C-rich tea from the tips of spruce needles. In 1535, when the French explorer Cartier became trapped in Canada during a severe winter, he and the men on his expedition were helped to survive by learning to make this brew. Similarly, missionaries who went to live with tribes in lower Canada and the northern Plains states were in danger of developing scurvy during the winter months. Some adapted to the native diet and brewed their tea from bark and needles recommended by the Native Americans and thus avoided scurvy. Those who persisted in drinking English tea got scurvy.

Missionaries who journeyed to Alaska faced greater difficulties. The Eskimo habit of eating raw fish struck them as heathen. In contrast, they scrupulously cooked their fish and tried to make the natives do the same. Cooking destroys vitamin C, so the missionaries' reward for their cooking zeal was scurvy. Fortunately, some of them learned that scurvy could be reversed if they ate the fish raw as the Eskimos did.

It's important to see how different people developed food habits and customs based on observation and ingenuity. Over centuries, they learned to meet nutritional needs with readily available foods or with materials we might not even consider food. Many of these customs, such as using acerola cherries and rose hips as sources of vitamin C, continue today in various parts of the world.

Lind to the Rescue

In 1747, Britannia ruled the oceans—75 percent of the globe. The empire's vast colonies stretched east to India and west to North America. But for the average British sailor, life was filled with perils. If he set sail on a voyage that kept him at sea for six months or more, scurvy could send him to a burial at sea. But some sailors did not get scurvy. Individual differences in vitamin-C requirement allowed some to survive, which must have seemed like a miracle at the time.

So great were the odds against survival that the captain of the 100-foot schooner *Salisbury* hired on a crew of 800 just to make sure that enough men would be left to steer the ship home after scurvy had taken its loathsome toll. The *Salsibury* had barely reached the Straits of Gibraltar when some of the men began to show symptoms of scurvy. When the captain ordered "All hands on deck!," the afflicted men couldn't move quickly. Physical symptoms were even more obvious. When sick crew members ate the hard, dried rations of bread and salt pork, their gums bled. They were vulnerable to all kinds of infection, from common colds to ulcerous sores that never healed. Blood vessels broke under the surface of their skins and appeared as tiny red fissures. The ship's doctor, a young naval surgeon, could not bear to stand by while the men in his charge sickened and died. Dr. James Lind set out to conquer scurvy.

One night as Lind left the officers' dining room to visit his patients in the mess hall, he noticed that ordinary sailors did not get any of the brussels sprouts and potatoes the officers received. Since officers did not get scurvy, Dr. Lind wondered whether the fresh vegetables protected them from the disease. Lind had read the accounts of Vespucci's voyage and the island of Curaçao, but being a scientist he thought it was something the sailors had eaten that cured them and not the island. Then the *Salisbury* came across a Dutch ship returning from Spain with oranges and lemons. Much to Dr. Lind's amazement, sick men who ate some of the fruit became well. Could something as simple as food cure this disease?

Lind decided to buy some of the fruit from the Dutch with his own money, and he set up an experiment that, although simple, launched modern research in nutrition. He selected twelve scurvy-sick sailors and divided them into two groups of six. Lind cooked all their meals himself to make sure each group ate an identical diet except for one item. Within six days, the men who had received citrus fruit recovered. For centuries, alchemists and witch doctors had boasted of magic potions that they claimed would cure scurvy; Dr. Lind's study provided a simple, indisputable answer to the problem. Unfortunately, his proposal that enlisted sailors get fresh fruit fell on deaf ears. The Royal Navy did nothing for nearly 50 years, although famed voyager Captain James Cook read Lind's work and prevented scurvy on his ship by putting in a supply of fruit. It wasn't until 1795— ironically, one year after Lind's death—that the Royal Navy ordered each sailor to be provided with a ration of lime juice, in addition to their daily rum, which is how the British sailors got their nickname "limeys."

What was in the fruit that prevented scurvy? Today we know it was vitamin C. But nearly 200 years had to pass before scientists were able to isolate pure crystals of vitamin C from lemon juice, and scurvy continued to claim victims. Many American pioneers died of it on their way west, before reaching California where the Spanish-built missions abounded with citrus trees. And in World War I, many troops of all nationalities died of scurvy.

Scurvy's Symptoms

In 1912, scientists started to refer to what they called the "scurvy vitamin" or "antiscorbutin" because it was "antiscorbutic" (prevented scurvy). In 1932, when the substance in fruits that prevented scurvy was identified, "antiscorbutic," was shortened to "ascorbic" and the new vitamin was named "ascorbic acid." This was shortened again to vitamin C.

Determining vitamin C's actual functions proved challenging because the symptoms of scurvy are manifested in so many ways. It was apparent that without vitamin C, the body literally falls apart: gums deteriorate and teeth fall out, blood vessels break, cuts don't heal, and infections set in. All this happens because vitamin C is required to make certain proteins. Protein is the primary component of the body. When you look in the mirror, you're looking at an amazing mosaic of protein. Hair, skin, eyes, muscle—much of you that shows and much of you that doesn't is made up of protein. The two dominant body fluids, blood and lymph, and the critical body tissues, heart and lungs, brain and nerves, are predominantly protein or depend on protein.

Many of the body's trillions of cells are constantly sloughed off and renewed. That takes a lot of energy and that's what some of the food we eat is used for. The process that maintains and renews the body systems by using energy and materials from food is called metabolism. Coordinating all the reactions involved in metabolism is every bit as complicated as launching a space flight, and the body does it automatically. If one nutrient is missing or out of balance, however, the whole system is affected. When a bricklayer builds a wall, he uses mortar in between the bricks to hold them together. When the body builds tissue, it uses a special kind of protein called collagen to make the cells adhere. Collagen is the body's connective tissue. As people age, collagen fibers lose their ability to hold the skin tightly together, so the skin sags and creases. And when the supply of vitamin C is inadequate, the body can't make collagen at all. Tissues that receive the most wear and tear, such as the gums, undergo rapid renewal and are the first to show signs of deficiency. Hence the bleeding and infected gums of the scurvy sufferer.

Collagen is also an essential part of strong teeth and bones, parts of the body once mistakenly thought to consist solely of calcium. Clinical evidence supports vitamin C's role in assuring the integrity of bones and teeth. For example, studies on restoring bone density in elderly women showed better results when the women took a multivitamin supplement with calcium than when they took calcium supplements. Very recent studies showed that monkeys on a vitamin C-deficient diet developed more cavities than those on a normal diet. Children who lack adequate vitamin C show less than optimal tooth and bone development, another example that calls to mind the scurvy-sick sailors who lost their teeth and experienced pain in their joints.

When you cut or burn yourself, protein tissue is destroyed. A minor cut usually heals, and within a week or two the skin looks as if it had never been cut at all. That's because the body's supply of vitamin C worked overtime to weave new protein fibers into place. In fact, people who have been severely burned or injured may require extra vitamin C to help their bodies heal.

Vitamin C in the Blood

Blood contains many kinds of proteins. Vitamin C helps these proteins perform their tasks, too, and if the diet falls short of vitamin C, these functions will suffer.

Antibodies are important blood proteins because they protect us from infection and disease. The immune system, including antibodies, is the body's main form of defense against the onslaught of the viruses, such as the one that causes the common cold, and against any type of invading bacteria. So many billions of harmful microorganisms surround us that our antibodies are constantly being used and must be renewed quickly. When vitamin C is insufficient, the immune system's ability to fight germs diminishes.

Capillaries are the tiny blood vessels that transfer blood from the arterial system to the venous system. Vitamin C helps keep the capillaries strong; without vitamin C they become fragile and hemorrhage at the slightest impact, showing up as purplish bruises or networks of tiny red lines just beneath the skin's surface. If you've ever seen a chronic alcoholic, you may have seen a face crisscrossed with these tiny red lines. Excess alcohol intake may not only increase blood pressure, but also interferes with vitamin C absorption. If capillaries are weakened, the combination may result in a change in facial color.

Vitamin C also takes part in the forming of *hemoglobin,* the most important constituent of the red blood cells, and helps the body to absorb iron, a key component of hemoglobin. It is the iron in hemoglobin that enables the blood system to carry oxygen to all the tissues of the body. In fact, it's the iron in hemoglobin that gives blood its red color.

When there's not enough iron, the blood can't carry as much oxygen. The result is weakness and fatigue.

A scurvy victim is deficient not only in hemoglobin, which carries oxygen, but also in adrenaline, a hormone that increases the flow of blood. Suppose you're at a movie and someone yells, "Fire!" You may find that you can run faster than you've ever run before. This is because of adrenaline. In a dangerous or tense situation, adrenaline is what gets your heart pumping faster, increasing the blood flow to the brain so you can think fast. It also gives you that extra surge of energy to either confront the situation or take off in the other direction, in what we call "fight or flight" response. Among its many other benefits, vitamin C helps to produce adrenaline. In fact, there is more of this vitamin stored in the adrenal glands than anywhere else in the body. Vitamin C's role in adrenaline metabolism may explain why British sailors with scurvy couldn't budge when the captain yelled, "All hands on deck!"

These are the functions of vitamin C that we know about conclusively, those that scientists have noted since the days of Dr. James Lind. In recent years, sophisticated technology has allowed scientists to study vitamin C in new ways and to develop new theories about its functions. Although these theories are still controversial, I believe they are worth discussing.

Vitamin C and Cancer

Vitamin C is one of a handful of nutrients in the body that are antioxidants. Some oxidation is vital—for example, oxidation helps break down food for energy—but if left unchecked, it can damage cell membranes and cause cell mutations. Since our intake of oxygen is constant, so is our need for antioxidants; they step in and save the day when the amount of oxygen by-products in the body gets out of hand. But in the process of protecting body tissues, antioxidants, such as vitamin C, are sometimes destroyed.

To see vitamin C's antioxidant properties in action, try

this simple experiment. Slice an apple in half, sprinkle lemon juice liberally over one of the halves, expose both halves to the air, and watch what happens. In a short time, the half not protected by vitamin C will turn brown, as a result of oxidation.

Bacon, pepperoni, and frankfurters contain nitrates and nitrites that the body may convert into cancer-causing nitrosamines. Did you know that nearly all vegetables and fruits also contain nitrites and have the potential to form nitrosamines? Unlike processed meat, however, fruits and vegetables such as broccoli, spinach and cantaloupes contain vitamin C. Emerging scientific research shows that vitamin C may neutralize the nitrosamines' carcinogenic potential. If one's intake of vitamin C-rich foods is less than adequate, consumption of meats containing nitrates and nitrites makes cancer of the stomach and the esophagus more likely. This is the hypothesis put forth by scientists who suspect a connection between vitamin C and cancer: namely, that vitamin C, like a football player blocking his opponent from making a forward pass, blocks nitrates and nitrites from forming nitrosamines and other cancer-causing agents.

Vitamin C and Smoking

It's been demonstrated that smoking cigarettes lowers vitamin C levels in the blood. Tests repeatedly find that smokers have lower plasma levels of vitamin C than nonsmokers. Theory has it that the vitamin C may have been spent defending the body. Although the vitamin-C depletion observed in smokers is small and considered inconsequential by some scientists, I believe it is indicative of vitamin C's important antioxidant function. However, if you smoke—and I hope you don't—please don't be foolish enough to think that taking vitamin-C supplements can compensate for all the damage you are doing to your cardiovascular system.

Vitamin C and Colds

If your vitamin C intake is inadequate, your body's immune system is not likely to work at its best. In recent years some scientists, led by Nobel prize–winner Linus Pauling, put forth the controversial theory that very large amounts of vitamin C prevent colds. Dr. Pauling's reasoning is based on the fact that most living creatures can synthesize their own vitamin C. When they do, it is in amounts far greater in proportion to body weight than the 60 milligrams recommended by the U.S. Dietary Allowance; sometimes six to ten times as much. Monkeys, who like humans can't make their own vitamin C, have a diet, whether in the wild or in captivity, that is much higher in vitamin C than ours. Thus, Dr. Pauling maintains humans have a better shot at staving off the common cold and other ills when our vitamin C intake is on a level with that of most other creatures. New evidence that gives some support to this was published recently by Dr. S. Boyd Eaton in a medical journal. Working together with an anthropologist, Dr. Eaton concluded that our prehistoric ancestors consumed an average of 400 milligrams of vitamin C per day. The researchers based their estimate on the vitamin C content of plants known to have formed a large part of the Paleolithic diet.

Of course the connection to contemporary people is tenuous and Dr. Pauling's theories are generally opposed by conservative scientists. And research on the common cold is difficult to conduct because of the myriad of cold viruses. But even though the body of research does not support the hypothesis that vitamin C can *prevent* colds, there is evidence that vitamin C reduces the *severity* of a cold. In any case, less-than-adequate intakes of most nutrients can make you more susceptible to disease.

What Happens When You Get a Chill

Imagine this. You're skiing hard and sweating profusely. After you make it down the mountain, you have to wait for your partner or for the next lift. A chill wind blows through your sweat-soaked garments. You may not realize it, but your antibody protection is taking a nosedive. And, if your tissue supplies of vitamin C aren't adequate, you are in a state of nutritional stress and may not be able to withstand cold weather.

Some recent studies of young skiers suggest that, when exposed to a sudden drop in temperature, the body's antibody level takes a dive. The antibodies most likely to be affected are those that are most capable of fighting the viruses that cause colds and flus. The body's ability to rebound quickly with new antibodies depends on its vitamin C level. People who have depleted their vitamin C supplies, whether because of poor diet choices, smoking, recovery from injury, or stressful situations may be more vulnerable to illness after being exposed to a chill than people with ample vitamin C in their systems.

Vitamin C Requirements

Most forms of life have some use for vitamin C, and nearly all of them can make it from a simple sugar called glucose. Cats, dogs, and rats make their own vitamin C. Only a few species lack the enzyme that would enable them to make this important vitamin: these are humans, apes, monkeys, guinea pigs, a bird called the red-vented bulbul, and the Indian fruit bat. There's an irony here because humans need more vitamin C than any other vitamin.

Some biochemists consider the inability of humans to make vitamin C an "inborn error of metabolism" and speculate that through mutations some humans are able to synthesize sufficient vitamin C in their bodies. Recall those sailors on da Gama's long voyage around the Cape of Good Hope; some survived scurvy and a few did not get it at all, even though two-thirds of the crew died from it.

You probably know people who catch cold very easily and others who never seem to get sick at all, or someone who complains of gums bleeding after flossing and brushing the teeth. The fact is that we still don't know all there is to know about individual requirements for vitamin C. It may very well turn out that the amount of vitamin C needed, like shoe sizes, varies from person to person. Some people may need more than others for their immune system and tissue synthesis functions. Despite differences in individual requirements, however, governments need to set standards to ensure the health of the general population. These standards have to satisfy the average person's needs.

In the case of vitamin C, scientists had to determine the minimum amount required to avoid scurvy. Research volunteers consumed vitamin C deficient diets to bring about scurvy. Once scurvy symptoms appeared, the scientists worked backward to calculate the lowest level of vitamin C that would prevent the appearance of the symptoms.

The absolute minimum requirement of vitamin C per day to prevent scurvy appears to be only about 10 milligrams. In order to allow for growth and maintenance of tissue and to compensate for losses in food, the Food and Nutrition Board of the National Academy of Sciences set the recommended daily allowance at 60 milligrams for adult males and females, since they recognized that the allowances may not meet the needs of people when they are sick, injured, or consuming a very poor diet.

Do We Get Enough?

Clinical symptoms of scurvy are almost unknown in the United States, which suggests that nearly everyone is somehow absorbing at least 10 milligrams of vitamin C per day. Despite the absence of clinical symptoms of this particular deficiency, however, a wealth of evidence from biochemial measurements and food-intake surveys indicates that many people in the United States don't get enough vitamin C to meet the standard requirement of 60 milligrams. Data from the Nationwide Food Consumption Survey, a gargantuan food-intake study by the government, found that 41 percent of the population did not meet the RDA for vitamin C. Of that number, 26 percent consumed less than 70 percent of what they needed. Other recent surveys show that getting adequate vitamin C is a problem for a significant number of teenage boys, young and middle-aged women, and the elderly.

Part of this shortfall can be attributed to choices. Luckily for us, many processed foods are fortified with some vitamin C and, unlike our more distant ancestors, we have citrus fruits available to us all year long. However, today we eat less than half as many melons, fresh potatoes, fresh cabbage, and fresh apples as did our grandparents. And so the vitamin C that we absorb from our food is less than it originally contained; part is destroyed during storage, processing, and cooking.

Now You "C" It, Now You Don't

Like other water-soluble vitamins, vitamin C in foods is extremely susceptible to destruction. Drying and canning, as well as cooking and storing, zap a food's vitamin C content. Commercially canned foods may contain more C than home-canned products if the fruits and vegetables reached the cannery fresh from nearby fields and were heated quickly in vacuum-sealed cans.

Prolonged exposure to air makes dried fruits and vegetables a poor source of vitamin C. Even fresh food can be risky. Spinach reportedly yields approximately 250 milligrams of vitamin C per 3 ounces. The measurement is based on samples fresh from the fields. But what happens after it's been trucked hundreds or thousands of miles to your supermarket? In one study, scientists found that fresh spinach had lost some of its vitamin C content by the time it reached the consumer. Unfortunately, there's no way to judge vitamin C content when choosing a bunch of spinach in the produce department. However, when spinach is picked and quickly frozen, sometimes more of the vitamin is retained—a case where modern food processing has improved rather than undermined the quality of our diets.

Vitamin loss doesn't stop when you get the produce home.

Such things as peeling produce, chopping it to bits, or boiling it in an uncovered pot in water that you later pour down the drain, all detract from the vitamin C available to you and your family. Further loss occurs if the food is prepared in a copper pot, mashed, left in a hot place, or exposed to the air.

Clearly, a high fraction of vitamin C is destroyed in restaurants and institutions where food is usually left on steam tables for hours. A study of five institutions, ranging from school cafeterias to hospitals, found that whipped potatoes had lost 36.2 percent of their vitamin C content after being kept hot for only one hour. Actual serving conditions may require even longer times on the steam table. Findings like these have raised serious concerns about whether hospital patients are getting the vitamin C they urgently need for antibody and collagen synthesis.

To get more vitamin C from produce, buy fruits and vegetables in small quantities and eat them fresh or steamed in a tightly covered pot. Make sure your supermarket keeps the produce on crushed ice or in refrigerated cases. Refrigerate all fresh produce immediately. Frozen produce retains vitamin C well if not allowed to thaw too long before cooking.

Vitamin C and IBD

Some people with IBD run the risk of not getting enough vitamin C. This risk comes from their need to peel fruit, the need to cook vegetables to softness, and the need to let fruits such as bananas ripen past the average. If limited variety and excessive cooking isn't enough, there's the increased need from drug use. We simply don't know what it is. But we do know that extra vitamin C, within reason, can't cause any harm and can do some good. Therefore, I urge people to strive for at least 250 milligrams daily. This means eating fresh, well-ripened fruit at each meal. I also urge you to read chapters Seven and Eight on supplementation.

The B-Vitamins: Of Mead and Meat

It is nightfall at a feudal manor somewhere in the depths of the Middle Ages. Seated around a table in the great hall, the lord of the manor and his knights quaff their cups of mead. They have just offered a toast to the lord's health. They have also just supplemented their diets with B vitamins. Mead, the beverage of choice in the Middle Ages, was made by fermenting honey. When taken straight from the hive, honey is mostly sugar and not much else. But thanks to the growth of yeast, fermented honey provided medieval folk not only with a good time, but with a rich source of B vitamins. Of course they didn't know about B vitamins, but they knew mead made them feel hale and hearty—even after the buzz was gone. It is probably because of mead that honey still enjoys a reputation as a health-giving food.

We are now in the heart of the African jungle of long ago. A swift hunter has just speared a lion. It is a muscular animal and its meat will be tough and stringy, except for the inner organs. While these are still warm, the successful hunter devours them. In his view, this organ meat will make him strong, for it will incorporate the spirit of the animal. In the view of modern science, he was ingesting such valuable nutrients as the B vitamins. The vitamins stored in the organ meat enable the hunter's body to tap into energy he didn't know he had. Thus, rituals evolved around the concepts of red meat and strength—rituals that have helped to shape the way we still prize that thick, juicy steak.

The Redneck

It's the summer of 1915. Imagine yourself working in the cotton fields somewhere in a southern state of the United States. More than fifty years have passed since the end of the Civil War, but the South is still devastated. People are desperately poor. Some of them have little to eat except for the corn they grind into meal; sometimes they add greens, rice, or sweet potatoes to accompany this meal.

Some workers are sitting under a cottonwood tree feeling weak and listless. Their foreman is cussing them as lazy good-for-nothings, as "shade-tree sitters." They hoist themselves up and go back to picking cotton. The hot sun caused their skin to burn badly; a condition that led to the name "redneck." Actually, the reddened skin was a sign that these workers and their families and thousands of others were very sick from a disease. In 1915, at least 200,000 Southerners were suffering from this affliction. About 10,000 died from it that year. What caused it? A vitamin B deficiency—but they didn't know it.

Pellagra: The Three Ds

The name of this vitamin-B deficiency disease is *pellagra*; it came from Italy where *pellagra* meant "rough skin"—the most striking characteristic of the disease was skin that first turned red on exposure to sunlight, then became dark and cracked. Other body tissues affected by pellagra include the digestive tract and the brain. A redneck might develop a sore mouth and tongue, inflamed membranes in the digestive tract with bloody diarrhea, mental disorientation, and hallucinations. Doctors nicknamed pellagra "the three Ds": dermatitis, diarrhea, and dementia.

No one was more concerned about the epidemic than Dr. Joseph Goldberger of the U.S. Public Health Service. As Dr. Goldberger journeyed south to find pellagra's cause and cure, hospitals, orphanages, and mental institutions had more victims of the disease than they could handle. Doctors then thought pellagra was an infectious disease, spread by germs in the midst of poor sanitation. But Dr. Goldberger had a hunch it was something else. When he visited an orphanage, he noticed that the infants and older children were healthy. The infants got milk regularly and the older children, who had to work, were given some meat. But children in the middle had neither milk nor meat. From this observation, Dr. Goldberger realized that pellagra was caused by an incomplete diet, rather than germs.

To prove his theory, on May 7, 1915, in the U.S. Pellagra Hospital in Spartanburg, South Carolina, Dr. Goldberger, his wife, Mary, and four assistants performed a heroic experiment. They mixed scalings of skin sores and intestinal wastes from pellagra victims with a little flour and swallowed it. Then they injected each other with the blood of a woman who had pellagra. None of them got pellagra, which was very strong evidence that the disease was not infectious. Thirty years were to pass before the workings of the B vitamins were understood. But in the meantime, people were taught how to improve their diets. By 1945, acute pellagra cases had disappeared.

Biological Teamwork

The name of the game is human metabolism. The winning team is the B-team—vitamins that control all human energy, whether that energy is used to build a bridge, pick cotton, or do a crossword puzzle. When just one B vitamin is missing from the diet, the body's pattern of metabolism is disturbed. Even if all the other raw materials are present, they cannot be fully used unless the B complex is present in its entirety. Cells may be unable to repair themselves with new protein, or cells may starve in the midst of adequate "fuel" because the fuel can't be burned.

The end result is tissue damage. As in the case of the pellagra victims, the damage shows up first in the parts of the body where the B vitamins are the most active. Both skin and intestinal cells are regularly renewed; this may be why diarrhea and dermatitis are two of the signs of a niacin deficiency.

In the body, vitamins cooperate with each other to do particular tasks, and the B vitamins are the epitome of teamwork at the cellular level. Thus deficiency symptoms overlap. Fatigue, for example, occurs when any one of the B vitamins is missing. Scientists only began to understand this biological B-team in the 1940s. We still don't know all the reactions that occur, or even among the reactions we do recognize, how all the transformations take place. We do know, however, that all the members of the B-team are essential for human growth, development, and metabolism.

The Body's Spark Plugs

In one sense the body converts energy the way an automobile does. In an engine, fuel in the form of gasoline combines with oxygen to make the car run. In the body, fuel in the form of food also combines with oxygen so the body can function. This is what metabolism is all about. In the car engine the mixture of fuel and air is ignited by the spark plugs at a very high temperature. In the body, a roughly analogous role is played by the B vitamins, which help oxygen to combine with derivatives of the food we've eaten. In this limited sense, the B vitamins together with various enzymes act as the body's spark plugs. First they help to break down food into its component parts, then to burn most of these components for energy.

Your need for energy is constant. Thinking, lifting an arm, even producing urine or sweat requires energy. We need energy not only to accomplish something, but also just to keep our body alive. But unlike the spark plugs, the B vitamins and enzymes do their jobs without explosions and high temperatures. After all, you couldn't very well walk around with a series of nonstop explosions talking place inside of you. Nor could the body's delicate organs tolerate excessive heat.

The B vitamins help regulate the release of food energy to the body at a slow, steady rate and at a relatively low temperature— 98.6° Fahrenheit. Instead of explosions, a long sequence of biochemical reactions occurs that enables the body to function as a "cool engine." The body synthesizes all the enzymes it needs to generate these reactions, drawing upon its biochemical pantry. But in order to operate, these enzymes require the help of B vitamins, which function as "coenzymes." And the body cannot make its own B vitamins; they must be supplied by the diet in the right amounts.

Let's return to the car analogy for a moment. Your car's fuel tank may be full of premium gasoline. But if just one spark plug is missing, the car simply won't run right. Here again, the workings of the body are similar. If just one of the B vitamins is missing or out of balance, the whole chain of energy-burning reactions is disrupted. You may have had plenty to eat, but if your B-vitamin intake was imbalanced or inadequate as in the case of the southern workers circa 1915, you won't have a normal amount of energy.

Meet the B-Team Members

At first scientists thought there was only one B vitamin. After much detailed research, however, they found, by the late 1920s, that vitamin B was not one, but several related vitamins. In 1927, a biochemist in Alabama suggested the term *vitamin-B complex*. At that time this family of vitamins was thought to have only three members. Today, when we say B complex, we mean the eight water-soluble vitamins that human beings require, along with vitamin C: thiamin, riboflavin, niacin, B_6, B_{12}, folacin, pantothenic acid, and biotin.

Let us sum up the characteristics they share before we look at them separately:

- They function as coenzymes for the release of energy from food and for nearly every cellular reaction in the body. Think about that. We have trillions of cells, and each cell undergoes a myriad of different biochemical reactions. In addition to being essential for normal growth and development, all the B vitamins are necessary for the maintenance of maximum physical fitness and healthy skin, hair, and nerves.
- Absence of any B vitamin for a sufficient length of time causes death.
- B vitamins are easily destroyed by canning, heating, milling, boiling, and other methods of food processing and storing. Some of these vitamins are also sensitive to light.

Rice Hulls and B₁

Thiamin was the first B vitamin to be identified. Sometimes called B_1, it's also known as the "morale vitamin." Thiamin was discovered when a food refining process led to a fatal illness. The Dutch, who conquered Java in the early 1900s, thought they were doing the native people a favor by building mills so they could have white, polished rice like the Europeans. However, the rice husk removed by the mills had been the people's only source of thiamin. Deprived of the husks, they developed a fatal illness called *beriberi*, meaning literally "I cannot." Weakness, lassitude, and muscle atrophy characterize the disease. Even in the early stages, the victims lack the energy to work.

Like the American doctors who later faced the pellagra epidemic of 1915, the Dutch doctors thought beriberi was an infectious disease. Vitamins were unknown in 1900. When a Dutch scientist fed an experimental flock of chickens the polished rice, they too developed beriberi. The scientist thought they had become infected. When his thrifty housekeeper supplemented the chickens' diet with rice husks, they became well. In 1913, the Polish chemist Casimir Funk, working in London, sucessfully repeated the beriberi experiment with pigeons. The vital factor was named "thiamine" (still often so spelled), and it captured the imagination of the world as the nutritional missing link, the vital amine! ("Vital amine" became vitamin, and today the word *vitamin* has come to stand for all of the organic minute nutrition factors essential to life.)

Later studies on people who volunteered to go on low-thiamin diets showed that after only ten days the subjects became depressed and irritable, couldn't concentrate, and lacked interest in their work. More critical symptoms followed within a few weeks. Normal health and morale returned when the subjects received thiamin. Thiamin helps break carbohydrates down into glucose, which is the brain's only source of energy. Glucose also converts to glycogen, our muscles' source of energy. Thus, thiamin deficiency affects both brain and muscle functions.

Today we eat many refined carbohydrate foods that are as depleted of thiamin as the polished rice of Java. Also, products high in sugar, fat, or alcohol demand thiamin from the body's limited supply in order to be metabolized. Yet they contribute no thiamin in return. They get a free ride, so to speak, at your body's expense.

Milk and B₂

B₂ or *riboflavin* was the next B vitamin to be isolated. This was extremely difficult, because riboflavin is so sensitive to light that scientists had to work virtually in the dark. Today we still contend with this problem. The clear plastic containers, in which many of us buy milk, allow light to diminish its riboflavin content. One of the chief sources of riboflavin in our diets, milk can lose 10 to 17 percent of this vitamin substance under the fluorescent light used in most supermarkets.

Breaking down food energy is riboflavin's chief energy role. The body burns primarily carbohydrates and fat for energy. Recent studies suggest that people who exercise heavily need extra riboflavin. During a marathon, endurance athletes usually burn more and more fats as the exercise duration increases.

Riboflavin can be found in every cell in the body. It is important not only for energy release, but for protein synthesis and many other reactions promoting the body's growth and repair. Unfortunately, the best dietary sources of riboflavin—milk, liver, and yeast—are not on most people's lists of favorite foods. Enriched cereals, lean meats, poultry, and eggs are good sources. Studies indicate that today many healthy, well-fed Americans rely on enriched grain products and supplements to help meet their riboflavin needs.

Lime Water and Niacin

Niacin is the B-team member that could have prevented many thousands of Southerners from dying or winding up in mental institutions or, at the very least, from suffering skin disease and diarrhea. Niacin is essential to biochemical reactions in the metabolism of carbohydrates, fat, and protein for energy. If it is lacking, the cells' energy pathways are completely blocked. Dependency on cornmeal triggered the pellagra outbreak in the South. Yet in many parts of Latin America corn flour is a staple and there is no pellagra. That is because it is common to soak the corn in lime water, a practice that makes the niacin in corn available to the body.

The body can also make niacin from the essential amino acid tryptophan, which is abundant in eggs, meat, and dairy products. Because these foods were found to cure pellagra, scientists thought perhaps it was caused by protein deficiency. Then someone cured pellagra with yeasts, and niacin was discovered.

Although pellagra is rare today, poor dietary choices can cause marginal deficiencies. Symptoms include nervous irritability, insomnia, digestive disorders, headaches, and a swollen, red, sore tongue. In children there may be weakness and poor growth.

Building Blocks and B$_6$

Pyridoxine, as B$_6$ is also called, plays the starring role in protein metabolism. It helps break protein down into its component amino acids. Then it works to build new proteins for the body from these amino-acid building blocks. It helps make the so-called nonessential amino acids, the ones that we don't need to ingest because the body is able to synthesize them. It also helps build hormones and red blood cells, and it acts as a catalyst to convert the amino acid tryptophan into niacin. As many as 50 amino-acid reactions require B$_6$.

B$_6$ also helps supply glucose to the brain and to the muscles. In case of deficiency, mental depression and muscle weakness can occur. Another job of this vitamin is to metabolize polyunsaturated fatty acids into components needed for cell membrane structure.

Processing food can drastically reduce its B_6 content. The classic B_6 deficiency story took place in 1951. A batch of commercial infant formula lost its B_6 because it was sterilized at an unusually high temperature. More than 300 babies across the United States began to have convulsions. Luckily, an official in the Food and Drug Administration realized what had happened, and the babies recovered with the help of adequate B_6.

We are not as restricted as an infant in our sources of food, nor are we dependent on others to select them. Yet many of us, unwittingly perhaps, tolerate diets dangerously low in B_6. About 75 percent of the B_6 in wheat is lost during the milling of white flour and is not replaced by enrichment. But how many people eat bread and cakes made with whole-wheat flour? Other processed or refined foods that we eat often contain less than half of the B_6 that was present in the food's natural state.

Certain kinds of medication, birth-control pills, excess consumption of alcohol, pregnancy and lactation, and old age—all may increase vitamin B_6 needs. Government surveys indicate that about half the population consumes less than 70 percent of the requirement for B_6!

B_{12} and Your Red Blood Cells

Vitamin B_{12} poses a special problem for strict vegetarians. As commendable as a vegetarian diet may be in some respects, there's simply no way to get B_{12} without consuming animal products. B_{12} is the only vitamin not produced by plants in any form. Even yeast, an excellent source of other B vitamins, contains no B_{12}. All animals have microorganisms in their intestines that synthesize all the B_{12} they need—all animals, except human beings. It's a persuasive reason for including some milk or eggs or a supplement in any vegetarian regimen.

B_{12} is so crucial to the production of red blood cells that lack of it leads to what used to be called "tired blood." People who have a condition called "pernicious anemia," which results from the lack of an intestinal B_{12} binding protein called "intrinsic factor," require a lifelong series of B_{12} injections. All body cells depend on B_{12}, particularly cells in bone marrow that produce red blood cells and those of the nervous system and the digestive tract. The vitamin is important for its role in the synthesis of DNA and RNA.

B_{12} deficiency symptoms result primarily in poorly formed red blood cells, indigestion, and diarrhea, and damage to the central nervous system. With lack of B_{12}, nerve tissue deteriorates, ultimately including the spinal cord.

The absorption of B_{12} requires a two-step process. A factor called "intrinsic factor" is released in the stomach. Intrinsic factor is required for B_{12} to be absorbed at the lower end of the small intestine. But what if the lower part of the small intestine is gone, as happens to some folks who have IBD? Your doctor can compensate for this with injections of B_{12} at appropriate intervals. Many people who have the ileum, or lower small intestine, missing, need B_{12} injections regularly and learn to administer them personally. It's no different than the diabetic who must take a daily insulin injection; except the B_{12} is not required daily. However, it is essential that you and your doctor discuss it regularly.

Spinach and Folic Acid

Unless you're a wheat germ, liver, and brewer's yeast fan or serve spinach and romaine fresh from the garden, you may be one of the many Americans with borderline folic-acid intake. People with IBD are especially vulnerable for folic acid deficiency. Azsulfidine, the most common drug used for IBD, reduces folic-acid absorption and can cause deficiency. Folic-acid deficiency is especially dangerous, and is easily prevented by taking a balanced daily food supplement.

One of the last B vitamins to be discovered, *folic acid* or folacin gets its name from *folium*, which is Latin for foliage or leaf. Folic acid was first isolated in pure form from spinach leaves. Like vitamin B_{12}, folic acid is essential for the formation of the nucleic acids DNA and RNA; cells cannot divide properly without it.

Although folic acid abounds in green vegetables and whole-wheat products, many people fail to get the daily requirement, even though it is only about one-half of 1 milligram. Why? Desserts, white flour, fat, and meat (excluding liver) figure heavily in the diet of many Americans, yet none of them contains much folic acid.

Folic acid helps break down the proteins that we eat into amino acids. It also helps the body turn some of those amino acids into new proteins, such as those used to build muscle tissue. Here it works together with vitamin C, B_6, and B_{12}—an example of teamwork in nutrition.

You can see how times of rapid cell division, like pregnancy, would increase the need for folic acid. Turning from the demand side to the supply side, folic-acid intake can suffer when total food intake is diminished; as in reducing diet or in alcoholism. Remember, too, cooking also destroys some of the folic acid in vegetables, as does storage in a warm place. So, store your vegetables in a cold place. And when possible, use the cooking water in a soup stock or sauce. It's a rich source of folic acid. Boiling vegetables excessively until "soft" destroys much folic acid.

Pantothenic Acid: The Everywhere Vitamin

Panto comes from the Greek word meaning "all," and pantothenic acid can be found in every cell in every living thing, plant or animal. All whole natural foods contain it, athough foods rich in other B vitamins, such as liver and legumes, are especially good sources.

Pantothenic acid works as a coenzyme with one of the master enzymes of the body. Together they collaborate in the workshop of metabolism, where food is broken down for energy and the elements are then built up again into complicated compounds that the body needs. Pantothenic acid also plays a role in fatty-acid synthesis, formation of red-blood cells, blood-sugar regulation, and the building of antibodies, nerve and brain tissue, and muscle tissue. Pantothenic acid, in many of its reactions, works together with riboflavin, niacin, thiamin, B_6, and several minerals.

Processing and freezing destroy this vitamin and lower the content in many people's diets. Foods such as corn flakes, precooked rice, sugar, and shortening contain little. Experimentally created deficiencies in humans produce symptoms such as fatigue, headache, sleep disturbances, stomachaches, and muscle cramps, but deficiences in a healthy population are practically unknown. Also, a deficiency would take months to develop. So, if you have a headache, don't jump to the very unlikely conclusion that you have a pantothenic-acid deficiency.

White Streaks and Biotin

Until recently, doctors had little concern for *biotin* because it was thought that the body could make it in sufficient quantities. But upon the advent of intravenous feeding in hospitals, patients developed severe rashes, depression, lethargy, and a loss of hair because the first formula diets did not include biotin. Now we know that although biotin is made in the intestines, we must also get some from our food.

Biotin is also required for releasing energy from carbohydrates and for the synthesis of glycogen for muscle energy, and of fatty acids, protein, and nucleic acids like DNA.

Hair is made up of protein. It's been found that hair growth slows or stops in people who are biotin deficient. In juvenile biotin deficiency, hair growth has been retarded; in fact, baldness resulted and hair was restored by supplementary biotin. In rare cases of severe adult biotin deficiency, hair has turned white; color returned when dietary biotin was provided. But it would take months of extreme deprivation for symptoms such as these to appear. Hair turning gray is a normal part of the aging process for most people and not the result of a biotin deficiency.

Biotin is most abundant in foods that are treasure troves

of other B vitamins; liver, yeast, egg yolks, whole grains, nuts, beans, meats, and dairy products are all good sources. An ironic note here: Many people think of a raw egg as being healthful, but actually raw egg white contains a protein that can bind biotin. Cooking egg white prevents this binding action, so go easy on the raw eggs.

B-Robbers: Empty Calories

Pretend it's lunchtime and you've stopped in a local restaurant. You have two choices: liver with brown rice sprinkled with brewer's yeast and steamed spinach, or a burger, fries, and Coke. Which would you choose? If you picked the burger lunch you're like many Americans. And like many Americans, you may not be getting enough B vitamins in your diet.

Here in the United States we have one of the best food supplies in the world. At any time of day or night we can select from thousands of food items. But in the absence of nutritional knowledge, too many choices can be a problem too. We can afford to be frivolous, so we often buy food for pleasure, not nutrition. We eat almost as a recreational sport. One result is overweight. A significant number of Americans lug around more fat than their bodies were built to carry.

But a more insidious result is borderline vitamin deficiencies, most notoriously of B vitamins. True, no one is walking around with pellagra. But many Americans place their health on a tightrope every day by barely meeting their minimum vitamin needs. Thiamin intake, for example, runs fairly close to the minimum. A fast-food meal of a hamburger, fries, and shake provides a large percentage of a day's calorie requirements but only 15 percent of the necessary daily nutrients. Fast foods and processed foods, because of their preponderance of refined ingredients, fats, and sugars, as well as their high cooking temperatures, won't fill the bill for the Bs.

We also put our health on the line when we consume

excess alcohol. Even if our bodies had enough vitamins before we drank, we might be deficient by the time we've sobered up. Alcohol requires B vitamins to break it down. But today's alcoholic beverages, unlike the mead (and the vitamin-rich beer) of yore, contribute no B vitamins to the body's pool. It uses up the body's B vitamins without contributing any in return.

Survey after survey finds that the intake of B vitamins is inadequate for many Americans, especially women, teenagers, and the elderly. While these people may not have deficiency symptoms, they may not be living up to their potential in terms of energy and achievement.

Water Vitamins and IBD

Vitamin C and all the B vitamins, except B_{12}, are absorbed throughout the small intestine. Even with 50 percent of the small intestine gone, you can absorb enough of these vitamins, with the exception of B_{12}, to get along. B_{12} requires injections. Once some of your small intestine is removed, however, you must get more vitamins from food or supplements to increase the total amount absorbed. For example, a 50 percent reduction of intestine should be compensated by at least a 25 percent increase in nutrients. (I estimate 25 percent and not 50 percent because the intestine is very efficient and can compensate to some extent for the loss in area.) But this is also complicated by the problem of diarrhea that decreases nutrient absorption. It's better to be "safe than sorry" and simply get more nutrients. It's a simple principle called "mass action" by chemists. Suppose you absorb 25 percent of the nutrients in your diet, and suppose you get 100 milligrams at each meal. In three meals that totals 75 milligrams. Now suppose you supplement with an extra 100 milligrams daily. That brings the level to 100 milligrams. It's a simple principle that works.

Folks with IBD are at serious risk for B-vitamin deficiency. Vegetables must be cooked longer and dairy products are often in short supply. You don't eat organ meats like liver and kidneys; indeed, you don't eat a lot of meat and for good reason. And today, who eats yeast? Add to a restricted diet the likelihood of some missing bowels, or chronic diarrhea. Then suppose you're on medication that destroys some of the B vitamins or increases the need. Supplementation is the answer!

Reread chapters Seven and Eight. There are many ways to supplement. We usually think of a "vitamin pill," but it can also be in the form of a food supplement. Either one works very effectively. Remember: a marginal B-vitamin deficiency can occur in only eight days. But it doesn't show up as anything significant—maybe tiredness, irritability, or some depression. Seldom does anyone even bother with doing something about them. It's better to make sure it doesn't happen.

CHAPTER EIGHTEEN

Macro Minerals: Sustaining the Skeletal System

Calcium, Magnesium, and Phosphorus

You don't drink milk? Neither do many Americans. Nor do billions of people all over the world. But in obtaining a regular supply of calcium, other cultures have some advantages that Americans generally lack. These differences make a bone-deep difference in the body's calcium balance.

Calcium is one of the most important minerals needed by the body in large quantities, and milk is one of the best calcium sources there is. But in most of the world milk presents some difficulties. Some nations simply can't spare enough land for grazing herds of cattle. For other nations, the problem is processing the milk. These countries lack the technology to pasteurize milk, and unpasteurized milk breeds tuberculosis. Even if people in the Middle East and Asia could get pasteurized milk, they would have trouble digesting it. They are "lactose intolerant" because their digestive systems lack lactose, the enzyme needed to break down milk sugar.

Many of these populations tend to be shorter in height than most Americans and Europeans, but they have well-formed, dense bones and as they age, they don't seem to be plagued with osteoporosis the way we are: As many as nine out of ten older American women show some evidence of bone disease, yet it is virtually unheard of in third-world nations. Following may be some reasons why. Many populations that maintain a healthy calcium balance without dairy products live in either tropical or semitropical climates. Lots of sunshine guarantees enough vitamin D for optimum absorption of the calcium they do get. Meat is a luxury for many third-world nations. People are primarily vegetarians, which bodes well for the bones. Meat intake seems to reduce calcium availability.

Carting around weight, even your own, while walking or jogging, is good for the bones. When was the last time you lugged water from a well or toted produce to or from a village marketplace miles away? People living in societies where even a bicycle is a luxury do plenty of that. In other words, some cultures, in which people never touch a drop of milk after infancy, add calcium to their diets and use it in ways that the average American would never dream of.

Limestone Tortillas

South of the border, Mexicans soak the corn that they use to make tortillas in lime water. In addition to processing the corn with lime water, a pinch of ground limestone is added to the tortilla itself. This practice dates back thousands of years. Mexicans eat tortillas with nearly every meal and are thus assured a reasonable intake of calcium. This system developed over thousands of years in an area where cattle weren't kept for milk.

How often do you eat Chinese food? Maybe once every few weeks if you live in New York or San Francisco, less often if you live in Omaha. But if you lived in Beijing, you'd eat Chinese food every day. Many of your meals would probably be cooked in the Chinese sweet-and-sour method. Dishes prepared this way rely on vinegar for their pungent punch. Besides providing mere taste-bud tingling, vinegar actually gives the meal a calcium bonus. The vinegar is so acidic that it partially dissolves any meat bones used to flavor the sauce. Calcium from the bones thus becomes part of the meal. Vietnamese cooking applies this same ingenious method for supplementing calcium otherwise lacking in the diet. After they eat the meat from a fish or chicken, the Vietnamese make a rich soup stock by cooking the bones for hours with water, vegetables, and rice to form a rich, thick liquid. What else do they add? Vinegar, of course. In Thailand, calcium carbonate is added to rice during its milling.

Europeans also developed many traditions for foods that are rich in calcium. No one is better than the Italians at making low-fat, high-calcium cheeses part of a meal. Many dishes, even desserts, make extensive use of cheeses like mozzarella and ricotta. Grated Parmesan and Romano function as tabletop condiments like salt and pepper. Throughout Europe, notably in France, meals invariably end with cheese and fruit.

Animal, Vegetable, or Mineral?

Minerals in the body were detected quite early—iron was found in the blood in 1747. But an understanding of the functions of minerals had to await a more sophisticated chemistry. Today we still use the term *mineral,* which was coined in simpler times when scientists thought they could easily categorize all matter. Back then a mineral was anything that was not animal or vegetable. Today we know minerals are part of both animals and vegetables. We used to think of all minerals as inert, like rocks. Today we know that's not accurate; calcium, to take one example, is extremely active in the body.

The name *calcium* comes from the Latin word *calx*, which

means "lime." This is also the origin of the word *chalk*. We come into contact with calcium daily as chalk, eggshell, seashell, bones, or limestone. All of these sources can fulfill the body's calcium needs, and in many cultures they do just that.

Boning Up on Calcium

On a dry-weight basis human beings eat a little over a pound—about 500 grams—of food per day. Nearly all of this food comes in the form of carbohydrates, fats, and protein, but a tiny bit, about 3 or 4 grams, ought to come from minerals. Much of that 3 grams should consist of calcium, which is what nutritionists call a "macro mineral." The body requires a total of about a dozen minerals, most in amounts so tiny that they are called "trace elements." Not so for calcium.

The U.S. Food and Nutrition Board estimates our daily calcium needs, depending upon our age, at 800 to 1,000 milligrams. Some scientists believe we need 1,200 milligrams and there are some who say women over age 50 should get 1,500! That's an average of about a gram per day, equivalent to about a teaspoon of limestone. By comparison, we need only about 300 to 350 milligrams of magnesium, 60 milligrams of vitamin C, and 18 milligrams of iron.

Why so much calcium? Calcium makes up from 1.5 to 2.2 percent of the human body. If you weigh 160 pounds, about 3 of these pounds are calcium. About 99 percent of this calcium forms the skeleton, the bones, and the teeth. A strong, well-developed skeleton fulfills a number of functions. It gives the body form, protects the brain, the heart, and other organs, and serves as an anchor for muscles that allow the body movements. Bone marrow, the tissue found in the center of the bones, is the site of blood-cell formation. Well-calcified bones are less likely to break or fracture. The remaining 1 percent of the body's calcium circulates through the bloodstream. But don't underestimate blood calcium because it's only 1 percent: it makes all our muscle contractions possible, including our heartbeat, which is the most important muscle contraction of them all. Blood calcium helps transmit nerve impulses; it plays a role in hormone function, and it's essential to the clotting of the blood. In fact, this 1 percent is so crucial to life that the body transfers enough calcium from the bones to the blood if it can't get it from the diet. Remember, the body is a fantastic survival machine.

The Calcium Balancing Act

You were probably told as a child to "drink your milk." Good advice. Now that we're grown up, no one tells us to drink our milk anymore. Why? Well, everyone knows that children build new bone as they grow. But most people think that once you're grown your bones stay the same—like the steel beams in a skyscraper. Nothing could be further from the truth. Bones are as dynamic as any other structure in the body.

The cells in the body, except for brain cells, turn over constantly—that is, old cells constantly die and new ones are formed. This process uses up some of the energy you take in from food. During childhood and adolescence rapid growth requires a rich supply of nutrients. Children need a growth "allowance."

In some parts of the body cell turnover takes place more quickly than in other parts. For example, you have a completely new intestinal lining every few days. This remodeling goes on more slowly with bone cells, but it does happen. New cells are formed; calcium supplied by the diet is deposited in the bones. If you looked at bone through a microscope, you'd see that it's structured so that most of the mineral crystals are close to a blood vessel. This helps the exchange of minerals and nutrients between bone tissues and body fluids.

All calcium from food first gets absorbed into the bloodstream after the food is digested. But only 1 percent of the body's calcium supply is supposed to be in the blood; remember? When there's more, say after you digest a glass of milk, a hormone stimulates the mineralization of bone. The extra calcium is removed from the blood and deposited in bone. Can you guess what happens when there's not enough calcium in the blood? Another hormone stimulates removal of calcium from the bone to put it back into the blood.

This is how the body maintains calcium balance. It's the same as if you kept a checking account with a constant balance of $1,000 and a savings account with $99,000. Any amount over $1,000 in the checking account automatically transfers into the savings account. But if the balance in the checking account dips below $1,000, enough funds will automatically transfer from the savings account to make up the difference. That's okay in a pinch, but if you keep writing checks and make no deposits, you will eventually deplete your savings. This is what many people do to their bones. And it's not just a matter of not getting enough dietary calcium. Other items in the diet compound the problem.

Protein: Tipping the Balance

Vegetarians, who get less protein on average than other people, do have an advantage: most meat eaters get excess protein, and excess protein increases calcium excretion. Meat is especially guilty of this. Given the typical American mania for meat, we've got a problem.

Except in North America, Argentina, Australia, and much of Europe, people eat small amounts of meats, if any. Chinese cooking is an example of a nearly meatless cuisine, but many other cuisines bear this out as well. Indian curry, Italian spaghetti sauce, and Mexican burritos all use meat more as a condiment to flavor vegetables and grains rather than as the main entrée. Much of our society, on the other hand, provides the body with large amounts of meat almost every day. We've also abandoned the European tradition of finishing a meal with cheese, which could help offset calcium losses caused by meat.

In societies with lower protein intakes, people get by with

less dietary calcium. Many people, especially Asians, seem to maintain an adequate calcium balance on as little as a few hundred milligrams per day. Actually, that's about as much calcium as many people get, despite the government's recommendations. The difference is that people in many other societies manage to utilize, more fully, whatever calcium their diets provide. By contrast, about 60 percent of our dietary calcium winds up flushed down the toilet. It never makes it to our bones. Other facts, like lack of exercise and exposure to sunshine, are most likely involved. But we do ourselves no favors with excessive meat consumption.

Magnesium

Calcium is not a solo performer in its balancing act. Like nearly all nutrients in the body, it's a part of a team. The other players on calcium's team are magnesium and phosphorus. In order for these nutrients to perform well together the diet must supply each of them in adequate amounts. Milk does this beautifully, but we don't drink much milk, and many of the foods we like to eat are low in calcium and magnesium.

Centuries ago an unknown Roman proclaimed the health benefits of "magnesia alba" (literally, white magnesium), the salts found at Magnesia in Greece. These salts, he said, could cure all kinds of ailments. Others found this to be so, and people from all over the Roman Empire flocked to Magnesia for the therapeutic salts. If they were suffering from a deficiency of magnesium, the symptoms would soon disappear. This was the first recognition of magnesium as a nutrient, and from this ancient spa the mineral got its name. A similar phenomenon occurred in 1618 in a village south of London called Epsom. The village water supply was found to have wound-healing properties and a laxative effect. The substance formed after evaporation of the water was called Epsom salts—magnesium sulfate.

In the technological world, magnesium is a light, structural metal used in airplanes and tools. In the biological realm, it's a central component of chlorophyll, the green pigment that enables plants to transform carbon dioxide and water into life-giving carbohydrates. Magnesium is also a major component of seawater, from which chlorophyll evolved.

The RDA of 300 to 350 milligrams for magnesium is 20 to 25 percent greater than what we actually require. The RDA is so high because magnesium is very difficult for the body to absorb. The human body contains 20 to 28 grams of magnesium—about 1 ounce. More than half of our magnesium remains in the bones; the remainder circulates throughout the body in the blood. The circulating magnesium supply is essential to health because magnesium is an important activator of enzymes, especially of those involved in energy production, working together with the B vitamins. Magnesium is also required for maintenance of bone structure, for protein synthesis, the transmission of nerve impulses, muscle contractions, and other important processes. Magnesium deficiency can cause weakness, muscle cramps, vertigo, twitching, convulsions, and muscle rigidity—all of which indicate its role in the neuromuscular system. Behavioral disturbances, such as depression, apathy, or delirium, are also part of the deficiency symptoms.

Magnesium and calcium are also involved together in blood-pressure regulation. Some people with high blood pressure seem to have developed it as an outcome of a borderline calcium-magnesium deficiency. It's one more reason why these two minerals are so important.

Although 60 to 70 percent of consumed magnesium is not absorbed, most of us seem to get at least a bare minimum. In our society, clinical magnesium deficiency can occur, however, usually from malabsorption, diabetes, protein deficiency, chronic diarrhea, alcoholism, prolonged use of diuretics, or gross malnutrition. Deficiency that comes to the attention of a physician can be easily cured. Borderline deficiency is sometimes found among adolescents and college students. Athletes, because of increased losses through perspiration, may also be at risk.

As one might guess, plant products, whole grains, beans, nuts, and vegetables provide the richest magnesium sources, but processing these foods causes great losses. There is little magnesium left in rice and white flour, and none in sugar, fat, or alcohol.

Diarrhea that is part of IBD interferes with magnesium absorption and can actually cause magnesium loss. To make matters worse, if you don't drink milk, or eat yogurt or cheese, your chances of getting enough are slim. Therefore, read chapters Seven and Eight on supplementation carefully with this in mind.

Phosphorus

Calcium and phosphorus together make up about three-fourths of the mineral content of the body. The amount of calcium present is twice that of phosphorus. A full 80 percent of the body's phosphorus interlocks with the bulk of the body's calcium in the bones and teeth. The remaining 20 percent circulates to every cell via the bloodstream, for phosphorus takes part in all energy-yielding reactions.

Phosphorus abounds in our diets. Meats, poultry, and fish furnish 15 to 20 times as much phosphorus as calcium; milk, cheeses, and green leafy vegetables are among the few foods that provide less phosphorus than calcium.

Meat, poultry, and fish are not the only popular American menu items that increase our phosphorus intakes. Soft drinks now occupy first place as America's favorite beverage, far outdistancing milk in all marketing surveys. A recent survey shows that we consume about 7.8 ounces daily per capita. This is a relatively recent marketing phenomenon. Only 50 years ago, soft drinks were a novelty or a special treat. Back then, this newfangled drink was frequently called by one of its chief ingredients—phosphorus. "I'm going to the drugstore for a cherry phosphate," Grandpa might have said on occasion. He may have had one of these drinks a month. Most adults drink two soft drinks a day; very little is consumed by children and the elderly.

The effect of dietary phosphorus on calcium balance is still under investigation. However, every clinical study done indicates that excess phosphorus causes calcium loss, which means that problems with calcium are compounded by heavy consumption of meat and soft drinks.

There's more. At least one other nutrient excess in the American diet contributes to a calcium crisis—fat. Excess dietary fat can bind calcium into insoluble "soaps" that are excreted. Again we can point an accusing finger at meat because of its high fat content. Societies that do well on very little calcium are primarily vegetarian and hold their fat intake to 20 percent of their calories.

So the next time you think you deserve a fast-food break, think of your bones. If you must have that burger and large soft drink, try to make sure you get ample calcium, too, or your bones will eventually give you the kind of break you don't want: the broken bones of osteoporosis.

Osteoporosis: A National Epidemic

Osteoporosis is becoming one of the most important health problems in our population. This crippling bone disease afflicts some 20 million people in the United States, most of them elderly women. Osteoporosis can disable and perhaps even shorten the lives of elderly people. Hunched spines, loss of teeth, broken hips, and other fractures result from this deterioration of the bones. It's estimated that 90 percent of all fractures in people over 60 are due to osteoporosis. Each year complications from hip fractures eventually kill 15 to 30 percent of all victims. Of those who survive, most are disabled and require nursing-home care. Experts estimate the cost of osteoporosis in this country at $3.8 billion annually.

Some loss of bone density occurs with age in just about everybody, but not everybody gets osteoporosis. The stronger the bones you've built throughout your life, the less likely you are to be incapacitated by losing a little bit. In fact, blacks, who generically have strong bones, seldom get osteoporosis at all. Diet appears to play a role in the development of this condition. A low calcium intake for most of one's adult years—a problem for most women—is thought by many authorities to be a contributing factor in osteoporosis.

The typical osteoporosis victim is a thin, elderly, white woman whose lifelong calcium intake has been marginal. To paraphrase the old saying, "the bone losses of old age so weaken the camel's back that it may break even without a straw being added." Because of hormonal changes, bone loss accelerates after menopause—one reason why women are more susceptible than men. But the trouble starts in adolescence when kids switch from milk to soft drinks. For girls the situation is bleak, even without the fate their hormones have in store for them; boys at this age are more likely to play active sports, and they haven't dropped milk entirely, both of which add to the bone mass that will carry into old age.

As girls grow up, the calcium crisis increases. On any day it is estimated that as many as 75 percent of all women do not consume the recommended 800 milligrams of calcium. A full 25 percent consume less than 300 milligrams. Soft-drink and meat consumption remain high. Little by little the body taps into the skeleton's calcium supplies. Some women already show a reduction in bone mass as early as age 25 and most show some decrease by 35 or 40. The calcium demands of pregnancy and lactation can further drain bone mass. If the mother's intake isn't enough to meet both her needs and the child's, nature will see to it that the child is provided for.

The degeneration of the jaw bone is a primary reason why so many elderly people lose their teeth. Once their natural teeth are gone, many older people can no longer eat fresh fruits and vegetables. Poor diet contributes to other health problems, especially in this vulnerable stage of life.

Trabecula bone, which makes up the vertebrae of the spinal column, also surrenders its calcium easily. By the time most women and some men are in their forties, they begin to experience occasional low back pain. Nearly all will attribute it to bad posture, a particular chair, their job, or middle age. Very few realize it may be a warning sign that the spine is weakening. If you were to examine the vertebrae in some of these people, you'd see that the bone has started to give way and sag in the middle. But this is just one possible cause of low back pain. The problem could also be a muscle sprain, kidney disease, or some other condition. Your doctor can help you determine the problem and whether osteoporosis may be a factor.

A woman's total bone mass at age 80 may be only half of what it was at 40. Much of the calcium that makes up the bone structure has been lost from the bone, released into circulation, and quickly excreted without ever being replaced. After being mined repeatedly, the bones are weak, brittle, and full of tiny holes, like an old dried-out sponge. Hence the name osteoporosis: "osteo" meaning "bone" and "porosis" meaning "porous"—literally "porous bones." Thus weakened, the spine may no longer be able to support the body's weight. The vertebrae collapse on each other and the spine curves into a hunchback deformity known as "dowager's hump." Without the support of the spine, the weight of the shoulders shifts forward, creating a stooped posture. The abdomen is also pushed forward as the spine shrinks.

As a result of stooping over and having compressed vertebrae, the osteoporosis sufferer loses height, anywhere from 2 to 6 inches and sometimes more. She has become the stereotypical "little old lady." Because weakened bones can no longer properly support the body's weight, spontaneous fractures may occur. We used to think elderly women fell and broke their hips; now we know that sometimes hips break first, then the women fall. The slightest fall can cause any osteoporotic bone to break, and it's not a clean break as in a healthy bone. Brittle osteoporotic bones shatter like glass, spreading bits and pieces into the tissue. Resetting the bone usually requires a skilled orthopedic surgeon, who may have to use devices such as steel pins or prosthetic joints to hold the bone together.

Although we once thought it was inevitable, now we

realize this disfigurement may be preventable. But for many people the realization comes too late. Osteoporosis *may* be stopped or even reversed; calcium supplementation, estrogen therapy, and exercise have all been shown to increase bone density in the elderly. Fluoride treatment can slow but not reverse the loss of bone density.

The total daily calcium intake required to maintain healthy bone density and calcium balance in postmenopausal women is now believed to be 1,000 to 1,500 milligrams. This is higher than the current RDA and much higher than the calcium intake of most women. Bone-disease experts recommend that all menopausal women take calcium supplements if their diets lack this level of calcium.

Exercise and Bone Density: Use It or Lose It

This may come as a surprise to you, but physical activity influences bone health. Extensive studies on astronauts and bedridden hospital patients all pinpoint inactivity as a chief culprit in bone loss. The pull of muscle against bone during exercise actually helps stimulate bone cells to reproduce. Thus activity spurs bone renewal and helps calcium retention. Weight-bearing exercise seems to be especially beneficial in maintaining bone mass. Gravity must play a role in this interaction. The body must pull its own weight against gravity to reap the greatest bone benefits.

Try to recall, for a moment, all those *National Geographic* photographs of people in nations where osteoporosis is not a problem. Visualize Egyptians carrying baskets and crockery full of grains or water balanced on their heads, or Chinese with wooden yokes, from which hang buckets of water or rice across their shoulders. Weight-bearing exercise is a way of life in other parts of the world.

Studies comparing runners to nonrunners, active and inactive college students, Norwegian lumberjacks and Norwegians who are not lumberjacks, all find that, given similar calcium intakes, the more active people have better bone density. In the United States, lack of exercise becomes part of a vicious circle. Many of us no longer have to strain to open the garage door. We don't even have to leave the easy chair to change television channels. To get our food, we need to do nothing more arduous than wheel a supermarket cart down the aisles. In fact, our lifestyle does not demand that we do any exercise at all, and many of us don't, even though we may wear jogging suits to the supermarket.

The damage to our bones from lack of exercise compounds the dietary deficiencies that erode bones little by little over the years. Once osteoporosis sets in, Grandma or Uncle Fred become even less active because their backs hurt. This only aggravates the problem. The skeletal system was designed not for easy chairs but for action.

Even in the aged, bones respond positively to exercise. In one study where the average age of subjects was 82, light to moderate exercise caused a 4.2 percent bone increase over 36 months, whereas the nonexercising group experienced a 2.5 percent decrease. So use it before you lose it.

Kidney Stones and Bone Spurs

No discussions of calcium would be complete without attention to these two conditions. Just because you have either condition does not mean you should deprive your body of its fair share of calcium.

Kidney stones are caused by multiple factors, including heredity and diet. Even with kidney stones, you still need to take care of your body's calcium needs. Obviously, if you're prone to develop kidney stones you should be under a physician's care; discuss your calcium need with the physician. People who have had kidney stones often tell me their doctor said, "Don't eat foods with calcium and don't take calcium supplements!" This advice flies in the face of experts who emphatically claim that people who get kidney stones still need calcium. It's just that they shouldn't take more calcium than they need.

Kidney stones are a significant challenge for people with IBD. This challenge comes from a "triple whammy": a side effect of commonly used medication; the production of too many organic acids that combine with calcium to form the stones; and dehydration due to diarrhea and the increased need for water. The stones aren't caused by too much calcium. People with IBD need as much calcium as anyone; it's just that they need to drink much more water than average, especially when they're taking sulfa medication. It calls for a serious discussion with your physician.

Another misconception is that calcium intake leads to bone spurs or calcium deposits. Researchers have found that these formations occur because of hormonal imbalances, and although spurs contain calcium, they are not caused by calcium intake.

Calcium and High Blood Pressure

There is much controversy in the scientific community concerning the possible role of low dietary calcium in the development of high blood pressure. Dr. David McCarron has shown that in some people with high blood pressure a low-calcium intake is a factor. His studies, and many others, show clearly that meeting the RDA in calcium and magnesium is essential to maintain normal blood pressure. The major cause of high blood pressure is, however, too much sodium and not enough potassium. But not enough calcium can be a significant contributing factor.

Calcium Supplementation

The use of lime in preparing tortillas and vinegar and bones in Vietnamese soup stock didn't become overnight culinary practices in their respective cultures. Over countless generations people observed that their children developed healthier bones, lived longer, and were stronger if they followed these particular dietary practices. They didn't know what calcium was, but without realizing it they were supplementing their diets with this important mineral.

Today we know approximately how much calcium we need and we know what foods contain it: dairy products, bones (in stews, soups, and canned fish), and dark-green leafy vegetables. Yet the typical American meal pattern may even increase the need for calcium as many medical scientists recommend. Our body's calcium balancing system can't cope with the protein and phosphorus excesses of the American diet. The solution then is simple. We should consume more high-calcium foods, or do as those in other cultures have done for thousands of years, supplement our diets with calcium and magnesium.

IBD

Calcium and magnesium are especially important minerals for people who have IBD. Absorption for either mineral is not efficient when things are normal, let alone when an intestine is inflamed or under the stress of constant diarrhea. During periods of diarrhea or ill health, these two minerals are likely to be forgotten. That's why I believe supplementations should be a serious consideration.

Another concern is lack of exercise. People with IBD should avoid becoming fatigued. Consequently, they don't exercise much, even though that's generally not the cause of fatigue when done properly. Combining a lack of exercise with the likelihood of poor dietary calcium and magnesium creates an above average risk for osteoporosis in women with IBD and possibly even men. It's a second reason why getting at least 800 milligrams of calcium and 400 milligrams of magnesium daily is so important. Read chapters Twenty-two and Twenty-three on stress and exercise for additional information on these two factors.

CHAPTER NINETEEN

Iron: The Red-Blood-Cell Mineral

A young woman makes her way through a public garden. She feels so tired that she sits on a bench to rest. Rummaging through her purse, she finds a mirror. Her cheeks and lips look pale, so she applies more lipstick and rouge. In a few minutes, when she feels rested, she will go on. This woman is not aware of it, but she probably has iron-deficiency anemia. Although earth's crust is 5 percent iron, iron deficiency is the most prevalent nutritional disorder in North America. The cast-iron bench on which the woman rests contains more iron than she will need for the rest of her life. From 15 to 25 percent of the population lack adequate iron. Yet iron is one of the most abundant elements on earth.

Swords, Nails, and Popeye

Thousands of years ago in ancient Greece, Jason and his Argonauts sailed in search of the fabled Golden Fleece.

To augment their daring and strength, these adventurers drank red wine mixed with the filings saved from sharpening their swords. The sword filings dissolved in the acidic resinous grape wine. They thought it was their weapons' savage power that lent their drink its strength. The real secret of the Argonauts was that they made the wine an effective iron supplement without knowing it.

Consuming enough iron has always been a problem, and like Jason, people have found imaginative ways to solve it. During Europe's Middle Ages, mothers would tell their daughters to pierce an apple with nails, remove the nails in a few hours, and then eat the fruit. We know today that iron from the nails leached into the apples, providing a ready source of supplemental iron. Wise mothers knew that it returned the rosy color to their daughters' cheeks and put back the sparkle in their eyes. In more recent times, during the cartoon animation heyday of the 1940s, the character Popeye the Sailor emerged. If you remember Popeye, then you recall his love, Olive Oyl, and his arch rival Bluto. Poor Olive was forever being chased and abducted by Bluto. She'd holler to Popeye for help but he was often too lethargic and lacking in stamina to respond until he gulped down a can of spinach. "I'm strong to the finish 'cause I eats my spinach," he'd sing, after subduing Bluto and rescuing Olive. Spinach is a plant rich in iron.

Popeye, it turns out, was a modern incarnation of a long line of mythological figures created to encourage children to eat foods that are good for them. These figures always drew their strength from particular healthful foods. Many of these myths evolved from the need for iron.

Iron as the Carrier of Oxygen

How does iron make us mighty? How does it help keep us bright-eyed, rosy-cheeked, alert, and energetic? There's no magic involved, just biochemistry. Iron transports oxygen, the leader of nutrients. Moving through the bloodstream, iron in the form of hemoglobin picks up oxygen in the lungs and takes it to every one of the 50 trillion cells in the body. Hemoglobin, part of all red-blood cells, contains a full 60 to 70 percent of the body's iron. Each molecule of hemoglobin can carry four molecules of oxygen. Iron is oxygen's faithful steed, its only carrier.

Cells rely on regular oxygen deliveries to help them derive the maximum amount of energy from the food we eat and from the fat our body burns in the absence of food. You could survive without water or food for several days, but go without oxygen for just a few minutes and the brain will suffer permanent damage; missing oxygen any longer results in death.

If your body lacks adequate iron, you won't have as much oxygen at your disposal. You won't be able to run as far or think as clearly. Not having enough iron prevents you from doing your best at anything, because oxygen is a key factor in everything we do.

Are You Anemic?

Your body, if it is normal, will make about half a billion new red blood cells while you read the last three pages of this book. But if your iron supply isn't up to par, the cells you make will be smaller, paler, and fewer in number than they ought to be. Like the anemic young woman in the beginning of the chapter, you too will look pale.

Red blood cells near the skin's surface create the rosy cheeks long associated with glowing good health. Folk wisdom instructed prospective husbands to look for rosy cheeks and red lips as signs of good health when selecting a mate. To enhance their marriage prospects some women relied less upon sticking nails in apples than upon simply reddening their cheeks and lips with cosmetics. However, cosmetics only cover the pallor of iron-deficiency anemia; they can't cure the weakness and lassitude that comes with it.

Without sufficient iron, the amount of work your muscles

and other tissues are capable of handling will diminish. New evidence indicates that, in some cases, chronic iron deficiency can also cause insomnia. In borderline cases, people with iron deficiency feel cold when other people don't. The brain, it seems, when deprived of its full oxygen supply, seeks to prevent the body from falling into the shallow breathing patterns of sleep. The heart has to work harder even in limited physical activity.

Your doctor can determine whether or not you are anemic by sending a small sample of your blood to a laboratory for analysis. The lab counts the number of red blood cells present in a smear made from the sample. Typical healthy red blood-cell readings range from 4.5 to 6.3 million per cubic millimeter in men and 4.2 to 5.5 million in women. Be aware, however, that you can be mildly iron deficient even if you have an adequate number of red blood cells that contain enough hemoglobin. Further blood tests may be needed.

Some of the body's iron is a constituent of myoglobin, a protein in muscle cells that provides a supply of oxygen for muscle metabolism. The body's second-largest concentration of iron is its reservoir in the liver, spleen, and bone marrow. These supplies may be depleted first without affecting hemoglobin. You may be low in iron reserves and not even know it. Poor growth in children, reduced physical fitness and work performance, lowered scholastic performance, reduced immunity to disease, digestive disturbances, and thin, brittle, or flattened fingernails can be symptoms of iron deficiency. Fingernails don't contain iron. They're made of protein. But they depend on good circulation and nutrients to make the protein; that's where iron comes in.

If iron deficiency becomes severe, all body functions eventually slow down and death ultimately results. This severe form of iron deficiency is rare. Nonetheless, anyone may be deprived of full vitality because of a borderline iron deficiency.

What You Get and What You Need

Iron plays hard to get. Very few foods provide substantial amounts. Foods that do provide iron can make it very difficult for the body to get at it. All kinds of biochemical barriers, especially in plant sources, can prevent absorption. Only 2 to 5 percent of the iron in vegetables, fruits, beans, and grains ever reaches the bloodstream. Iron in meat has a better chance of making it; about 15 to 35 percent can be absorbed, provided it's not blocked by other components of a meal, such as the tannins in tea and coffee and the phosphates and carbonates that give soft drinks their fizz. The U.S. Food and Nutrition Board has tried to overcome these barriers by setting the recommended dietary allowance upon iron.

Iron is so crucial to our ability to use oxygen that the body recycles iron from old blood cells to new. Every day the body typically recycles 30 to 40 milligrams. The only way a substantial amount of iron leaves the body is through bleeding. Losses in urine, sweat, and sloughed-off skin, hair, and nail cells account for only 1 milligram per day; menstruating women pose a special situation we'll address later.

This 1 milligram is the basis for determining our minimum daily needs. To replace it, the iron recommendation for adult men, infants, children ages 4 to 10, and postmenopausal women is 10 milligrams per day, of which about a tenth is absorbed. Since rapid growth always requires extra iron, the recommendation for children 6 months to 3 years old is 15 milligrams, and for a teenager it's 18 milligrams—the same as the requirement for women of childbearing age. That's not much. If you took a pinch of sugar from the bowl, you'd have much more than 18 milligrams of it between your fingers. And there are various ways to get this much iron.

To get 18 milligrams of iron the diet must provide at least 8 milligrams of iron for every 1,000 calories. But the diets of many people have become so diluted by processed foods that for every 1,000 Calories we now average only about 6 or fewer milligrams of iron. No wonder that, according to nutrition surveys, nearly 60 percent of us don't get enough iron. Women, children, and teenagers have the biggest gaps between their iron needs and actual intakes.

A Special Problem for Women

Iron deficiency occurs for three basic reasons: lack of iron in the diet, poor absorption of the iron we eat, and loss of blood. The first two are everybody's problem. But loss of blood is mainly a woman's problem, except for bleeding associated with intestinal disorders; people with these medical conditions should be carefully monitored by a doctor. But most healthy menstruating women are on their own when it comes to nutrition.

From infancy up to adolescence boys and girls share identical needs. But, once hormonal changes occur, their nutritional paths diverge, not to meet again until the last leg of life's journey—old age. For iron, the divergence occurs around age 19. Once a young man has developed all the blood cells and new muscle tissue for his adult body, his iron needs drop from the adolescent high of 18 milligrams daily to a maintenance level of 10 milligrams. And there he stays for the rest of his life.

For women, however, it's another story. Once menstruation begins, iron needs remain at a high of 18 milligrams per day from puberty until menopause. A woman's diet must replace the iron she loses every month in menstrual blood. If her intake does not balance out her losses, a deficiency develops.

Most women in the United States live on 1,500 to 2,000 Calories a day. If the average American diet provides only 6 milligrams of iron per 1,000 Calories, then American women wind up with only 9 to 12 milligrams of iron daily, instead of the optimal 18. Yet most women find it difficult to maintain their ideal weight even at these low Calorie levels. The reason? Not enough exercise and too many empty Calories from such treats as chocolate-chip cookies and potato chips. As iron-poor junk foods predominate in the diet, women may become iron deficient and too tired to exercise. Without enough activity to burn all the Calories they eat, they gain weight, in response to which they eat even less and further reduce their intake of iron.

Think about it for a moment. Just to wash dishes a woman once had to chop firewood, fetch water from a well or pump, build a fire to heat the water, and then wash the dishes—along with churning butter, kneading bread dough, and hand washing clothes. Today dishes and laundry are loaded in their respective washing machines and bread and butter are picked up at the supermarket. Even the electric typewriter saves a secretary 3 Calories each day.

Modern conveniences save time but, unfortunately, also reduce the occasions for exercise. In order not to become overweight, women have unknowingly adjusted their food intakes downward. But even if women ate twice as much as men do, they might still be deficient in iron unless they ate the right foods. Studies analyzing the diets of the U.S. Olympic ski teams found that female skiers often consumed more than 3,000 Calories a day, but did not always get 18 milligrams of iron. They ate too many "empty Calories" —foods that provided Calories but few vitamins and minerals.

When women whose iron intakes are marginal become pregnant, disaster looms, because nature gives the baby priority for all nutrients. Iron is needed to build the placenta as well as the unborn child's blood cells, muscles, enzyme systems, and other organs, such as the spleen and liver. The baby's iron needs are enormous during those first few months, and the mother may not have enough for two. Many obstetricians now include iron in a separate prenatal supplement program. In fact, iron is such a problem for today's American women that the U.S. Food and Nutrition Board recommends that *all* pregnant and nursing women take an iron supplement.

Eating Natural Foods

Now let's go back to the anemic young woman who opened this chapter. Let's say she realizes that she's tired and pale because she needs more iron. "How do I get it?" she wonders.

First of all, she could try eating more natural foods. Minerals may be lost in processing. Iron-deficiency anemia has become increasingly common as foods we eat are more and more refined. For example, milling cereals can remove 75 percent of the iron content from the grain. Second, she could increase her ability to absorb iron by adding vitamin C to the meal. The absorption of iron from vegetables, normally poor, improves when they are consumed with sufficient vitamin C. Third, unless she is a vegetarian, this woman could consider eating certain meats that contain far more iron than grains or vegetables do. At best, a half cup of cooked spinach provides only 2 milligrams of iron and kale provides only 0.7 milligrams. A slice of whole-wheat bread provides 0.8 milligrams. Remember, a woman of child-bearing age needs 18 milligrams per day. That's 13 cups of cooked kale or more than 22 slices of whole-wheat bread. Of course many other plant sources, like beans, can provide small amounts too, and it all adds up. But there's no denying it: meat is the best food source of iron.

Since animals, like humans, need a certain amount of iron to live, meat provides a richer source of iron. Not all meat contains equal amounts; much depends on how the animal was reared and slaughtered. Our food supply has changed greatly in the last 20 years or so. Now much of the iron-containing blood is removed from meat and sold for use in by-products. Still, a large hamburger provides 3 milligrams of iron, a little better than spinach. It's downhill from there, though, with rib roast, chicken, and fish all providing 1 to 2 milligrams per serving.

The secret is a particular kind of meat—the liver. Time was when the butcher threw in a slice of liver for every piece of meat you bought. In those days families ate liver once or twice a week. Liver is the body's iron supply depot and that goes for animals, too. A slice of calves liver contains 12 milligrams of iron. Pork liver provides 24 milligrams. One drawback is that liver carries a heavy price tag in terms of cholesterol, and few people with IBD are likely to eat liver.

Another factor reducing iron intake is that we no longer cook in old-fashioned cast-iron pots and pans. These actually add significant quantities of iron to the foods cooked in them. But today we prefer color-coordinated enamel, aluminum, or nonstick-coated cookware.

So if the young woman upped her caloric intake and ate several cups of cooked leafy green vegetables a day, one serving of liver, lots of beans and whole grains, along with vitamin C, and cooked it all in cast-iron pots and drank no coffee with her meals, she might be able to rev up her system with the iron she needs.

She might be able to eat like this—but can you? It doesn't hurt to try, but remember, a supplement with both iron and vitamin C can provide nutritional insurance in case your diet falls short of your intentions.

IBD: Special Challenges for Iron

IBD presents a special challenge when it comes to getting dietary iron. During periods of flare-ups, most people with IBD don't eat red meat. And many don't eat it even when they're feeling good. Other rich sources of iron—clams, oysters, and mussels—are unlikely to be eaten because they're often listed as causes of flare-ups. It all builds a good case for food supplements, especially a supplement that provides iron.

A second reason for IBD sufferers to supplement with iron is diarrhea. When diarrhea persists, poor nutrient absorption follows. To make matters worse, any intestinal bleeding adds iron loss to poor absorption. Intestinal bleeding is a constant companion of many people with IBD. Getting the RDA of iron each day is essential.

CHAPTER TWENTY

Trace Minerals: A Little Goes a Long Way

A man in New Jersey loses his ability to taste and smell. A woman in China has hands crippled with painful swollen joints resembling rheumatoid arthritis. A child on the island of Crete is born mentally and developmentally disabled. What do these afflicted people have in common?

Each is deficient in an essential mineral needed by the human body in minute amounts. The amounts are so small, in fact, that early biochemists working without today's advanced techniques could barely discern them in tissue samples. Hence, the biochemists called them trace minerals when they did detect their presence.

Our requirement for trace minerals ranges from milligram amounts for iron and zinc down to micrograms—that's one millionth of a gram—for minerals such as selenium and chromium. In a 150-pound body, the total of *all* trace elements is 25 to 30 grams—about 1 ounce—compared to over 1,000 grams of calcium and about 30 grams of magnesium.

Trace minerals are among the pieces most recently fitted

into the human nutrition puzzle. The essential functions of some were discovered as recently as the 1960s and 1970s. We don't know enough about some of these trace minerals for the government to establish a recommended daily allowance specific for age and sex. That refinement awaits future decades. However, scientific understanding of some trace elements has enabled the government to at least set "safe and adequate ranges" for them. We will look at these trace elements and at zinc in this chapter.

Blue-Flour Tortillas

Most of us are within convenient distance of a Mexican restaurant. There we might savor tortillas, a chewy, crepelike pancake used in older times as an edible utensil made from corn flour. Our tortilla would be cooked to a nice, light, golden brown the way we like them. But, in the southwestern part of the country, people of Mexican extraction prepare "blue-flour" tortillas, following the custom that originated in old Mexico. A blue-flour tortilla starts out like any other tortilla, but before cooking it, a Mexican dusts each side with ashes saved from burning the corn leaves. When the tortilla is cooked, the ash gives it the bluish tinge.

When traveling in the Southwest, I wondered why people with a limited diet would purposely make a staple food look less appealing. I've always believed these specialized food patterns are influenced by such scarcity, religious customs, and nutritional advantage. As a nutritionist, I had a hunch that the ash on the tortilla contributed to health.

Tortillas are made from corn kernels. In subsistence societies, such as those of the Native Americans and Mexicans, nothing is wasted. The corn cobs are used as miniature fuel logs to boil water and cook. Meanwhile the leaves, stems, and stalks of the corn plant are reduced to the ash, which I believe is the Mexican family's trace-mineral supplement. The ash contains the minerals the corn plant absorbed from the soil. These include calcium, iron, manganese, and other elements, ranging from zinc to copper. The blue cast of the tortilla comes primarily from oxidized copper, the color of an old copper kettle. In addition to the ash, the Mexican homemaker also adds a pinch of limestone to each tortilla, which provides her family with calcium and magnesium.

Iodine: Seaweed and Burnt Sponge

Calling someone a cretin is an insult implying stupidity. But the term derives from a specific form of mental retardation called cretinism. This was a tragedy that befell many children born long ago on the island of Crete, where iodine-deficient soil prevails. Cretinous children have underdeveloped thyroid glands. Their short life spans were lived as mentally disabled, partially deaf dwarfs as a result of a deficiency of iodine in the mothers' diet. The children were deficient in iodine before birth, while nursing, and then after going on to eat table food.

In adults, this iodine deficiency manifests as goiter, a grotesque swelling of the neck. If unattended in its early stages, a goiter will continue to grow. Eventually it can become large enough literally to choke the iodine-deficient person to death. Goiter was known in China as early as 3000 B.C. and has afflicted people throughout the world. One of the saddest aspects of iodine deficiency, whether it occurs as cretinism in newborns or as goiter in adults, is that prevention or cure is so simple.

If all the other nutrients involved in metabolism are thought of as a vast symphony orchestra, iodine is the conductor. It operates by forming two key hormones in the thyroid gland—thyroxine and triiodothyronine—which together are key players in the regulation of metabolism. These hormones are required for growth, reproduction, nerve formation, mental health, bone formation, protein synthesis, and all aspects of energy metabolism. Without iodine in the diet, none of these activities can take place properly.

Our RDA for iodine is only 150 micrograms. This is such

a small amount that the weight of iodine an adult woman requires for a whole year would amount to only 54 milligrams—just enough to cover the period at the end of this sentence. Because it's so critical, the iodine RDA was set at double our minimal needs to provide a margin of safety.

When there's not enough iodine in the diet, the whole system slows down and the person becomes listless and inactive. As the thyroid gland strains to catch any bit of iodine the blood might contain, it swells. The swelling increases to form the goiter. Unfortunately for people, plants don't require iodine for growth. So unlike other minerals, iodine is present in plants only if they happen to grow in iodine-rich soil.

Interestingly, the sea abounds with iodine. In many cultures where goiter and cretinism may have been endemic at one time, someone, no doubt, noticed that those who ingested ample seafood and sea plants thrived. Thousands of years ago, the Chinese effectively treated goiter by feeding seaweed or burnt sponge to the stricken. In fact, because the same methods were used by the Incas of Peru, some anthropologists theorize that the Incas are descendants of the same people. Greek and Egyptian fishermen also consumed the ash from burnt sponge to avoid the symptoms of iodine deficiency. Today dried seaweed, shellfish, and other types of seafood continue to be principal sources of iodine for many cultures.

In the United States, iodine deficiency is a thing of the past. In 1918, when men drafted for World War I were examined, it was discovered that goiter was a problem only in certain low-iodine regions such as the Great Lakes states and the Pacific Northwest. Scientists further realized that farm animals from goitrous regions also suffered from deficiency symptoms. Many studies were done, and by the 1920s, simply iodizing common table salt solved the problem. Also, our modern food-distribution system ensures that no one is dependent solely on locally grown produce. Thus we have eliminated the "goiter belts" in this country.

In fact, because of our increased intake of salt-processed

foods as well as iodine's use in animal feed and food additives, our intakes have skyrocketed in the last few decades. A typical fast-food meal provides three times the RDA of iodine because it's so excessive in salt. Some scientists fear we may even be approaching toxicity levels.

Selenium: Tea and Locoweed

About 2000 years ago in parts of China, people learned to brew a tea from a plant called astragalus. The tea wasn't a refreshment, it was medicine. Drinking the tea prevented or cured Kashin-Beck disease, which caused swollen joints and complete disintegration of cartilage. Kashin-Beck disease is a sign of selenium deficiency. China's soil, even today, has the world's lowest selenium levels.

Plants of the genus Astragalus are known throughout the world as selenium-accumulator plants. They can extract any bit of available selenium from the soil. In fact, where soil selenium levels are high, the plants accumulate so much that they become toxic. In the western parts of the United States, for example, a type of this plant is called locoweed, because when grazing livestock consume it, they develop a disorder known as "blind staggers" and eventually die. Yet in parts of China, the soil is so low in selenium that similar plants supply just enough to meet people's needs.

But China is a vast nation with a billion people and, unfortunately, not all of them were aware of, or had access to, astragalus tea. In 1979, after millennia of intensive agriculture, the selenium in some rural areas was so depleted that epidemic numbers of local people, especially children and women of child-bearing age, began to develop deficiency diseases. The situation was desperate and the Chinese government turned to scientists throughout the world for help. In fact, I was present when another scientist showed a physician an X ray of a Chinese child's hand. "My gosh, it's a perfect case of juvenile rheumatoid arthritis," the doctor exclaimed. He was quite surprised when he learned it was Kashin-Beck disease. In addition, another disorder emerged: Keshen disease, which causes fatal deterioration of the heart muscles.

For a four-year period, the Chinese government ordered that nearly 40,000 children be fed selenium orally, and the death rate was greatly reduced. Many scientists diligently followed the proceedings since it would be impossible to induce similar conditions clinically on volunteers. Tragic as nationwide epidemics are, they have one silver lining: They usually help scientists discover something new and important about human health. This was just as true for selenium in 1979 as it was for niacin in the 1920s.

Scientists now know that selenium works with vitamin E to help protect cell membranes from oxidative damage caused by harmful chemicals. Among these potentially harmful chemicals are the so-called free radicals or peroxides, similar in action to the ones used in some laundry bleaches. Free radicals can be a result of natural events, such as the cosmic rays that bombard our planet or of artificial conditions, such as auto exhaust fumes and factory smoke.

In animals, lack of selenium weakens blood capillaries, causes muscular dystrophy, and damages hearts. Of these, only the heart problem has been found in selenium-deficient humans, along with the arthritislike Kashin-Beck disease.

It may be a coincidence that Americans living in states with high levels of soil selenium show lower death rates for some types of cancer than those in other states. But it is important to keep in mind that these people are not consuming excessive amounts of selenium, or they would have a high death rate from selenium overdoses, because selenium can be an extremely toxic mineral in large doses.

Dietary selenium in North America is sufficient to avoid serious deficiencies. Soil and water levels vary across the North American continent, but the average American's selenium intake is believed to be 100 micrograms per day. The government's current safe and adequate range is set at 50 to 200 micrograms per day.

However, studies by Dr. Julian Spallholz showed that

only 60 percent of ingested selenium is absorbed. This may indicate that, although American intakes may be sufficient to prevent deficiency disease, they may be inadequate to provide the full benefit of selenium's antioxidant protection.

Seafood, meat, and whole grains can be good selenium sources. If you choose to supplement your diet with selenium, remember that a little bit goes a long way. The total selenium in your body would fit on a match head. As small an amount as 2.5 milligrams a day can be toxic; this mineral, while important, shouldn't be taken to excess.

Copper: A Penny in the Pickle Jar

There's an old saying about putting a penny in the pickle jar. Pickles were homemade in the old days. Every homemaker wanted to put up pickles that the family would enjoy and that might win a ribbon at the county fair. The penny helped keep the pickles just the right shade of green. It was supposed to be healthy, too. And it was.

Copper is the element at work here. As the copper in the penny began to dissolve in the pickling solution, it turned blue-green, just as the copper in the corn ash turns the Mexicans' tortillas blue. Both the penny and the ash are a means of supplementing the diet with copper.

All plants require copper. In humans, copper helps the body produce the hemoglobin in red blood cells. It functions in many important enzyme reactions and thus also takes part in energy metabolism. We don't need very much copper, however. The government's safe and adequate range is 2 to 3 milligrams per day. An adult body contains only 75 to 150 milligrams, which is less than you'd find in a penny. In fact, a penny probably contains enough copper to last a year.

As a rule we absorb nearly half the copper we consume. Interference by high levels of zinc in the diet or extensive use of antacids leaves us with less. Like magnesium, copper is also lost in perspiration. Some scientists argue that, when a person perspires profusely, say during heavy exercise or extreme heat, too much copper may be lost. Copper deficiencies, when they do occur, show up as pallor, convulsions, poor growth, scurvylike sores, and prematurely gray hair. High doses of copper can relieve these symptoms, but not everyone with prematurely gray hair has a copper deficiency; otherwise, people could just take copper supplements and no one would ever go gray.

Although copper deficiencies are rare so far, the processed foods that form an ever-increasing proportion of our diets are poor sources. Copper is present with other minerals in all natural foods. Some of the richest sources are meats, beans, shellfish, nuts, and cocoa. People may inadvertently get a copper boost from copper cooking utensils, water pipes, or the machinery used to pasteurize milk.

A well-balanced multivitamin-multimineral supplement can also ensure that intake is adequate. But copper bracelets, although possibly attractive jewelry, are worthless for copper supplementation—even if they do turn your arm green.

Without Zinc, It Stinks

In the early 1970s, a man who owned a very profitable pizza parlor in New Jersey was disturbed when the pizza aroma he loved so much suddenly became disgusting to him. As days went by, the scent of his product became more and more obnoxious until he could no longer tolerate it. He sold his pizza parlor and tried to find another way to earn a living. But by then other familiar smells and tastes began to take on different characteristics, some distinctly nauseating. Doctor after doctor failed to find anything wrong. Finally his case was referred to the National Institutes of Health. There, Dr. Richard Henkin identified the problem as zinc deficiency and treated it accordingly. Henkin named this disorder, wherein the ability to smell and taste becomes confused, "disgusia." Zinc deficiency may also be the culprit, he found, in a variation he called "agusia." In this form, the individual loses the ability to taste or smell anything.

These discoveries catapulted zinc into new prominence. Barely ten years had passed since zinc was found to be essential to human health. This discovery, in the 1960s, occurred when areas in the Middle East were found to have a high incidence of people with dwarfism and undeveloped sexual organs. In classic nutrition studies, young men with these disorders grew in stature and developed normal sexual characteristics after being provided with zinc supplements. If zinc deficiency persists too long, however, it cannot be reversed; the individual must go through life without ever reaching full physical maturation.

From these studies scientists concluded that zinc is essential to metabolism and protein synthesis and is especially important in growth and development. Thanks to the work of Henkin and others, we now know that zinc is involved in most enzymes vital for the growth and metabolism of certain cells and tissues. In fact, no other nutrient in the body is part of so many enzymes. Only 2 grams of zinc are found in the entire body, but they really get around.

Zinc is one of the many nutrients necessary for the immune system. It may help prevent infection by its role in regulating the functions of some white blood cells. White blood cells are one of the body's important lines of defense against invading bacteria or viruses.

A study by Dr. George Eby indicates that large amounts of zinc help reduce the severity of a cold. Although the reason is not clear, it could be connected with zinc's role in the immune system. Beware, though: large amounts of zinc can cause other problems and should be used with a doctor's guidance.

In some cases, one of the symptoms of zinc deficiency is poor wound-healing. This involves zinc's role, together with vitamin C, in the synthesis of protein, particularly of collagen, the protein that forms the skin's connective tissue. When a wound heals, the body has to make extra collagen and other proteins to replace what was lost. Without adequate zinc, this takes much longer. Zinc ointment has been found to help cuts heal. One may speculate that applying zinc to the damaged cells may help the body fight infection as well as help repair the wound. A secondary effect is from the zinc salts, which actually kill the viruses.

Zinc is also important to vitamin-A metabolism. Zinc deficiency can lead to lower vitamin A levels in the blood, just as a deficiency of vitamin A itself would. Vitamin A is also responsible for the health of skin cells. Zinc's connection to vitamin A led scientists to investigate a possible role for zinc in relieving some skin conditions. Zinc has an important role in a number of conditions, including alcohol-induced liver disease, surgery, burns, sickle-cell disease, and cystic fibrosis.

The adult RDA for zinc is set at 15 milligrams. The body actually needs 2.5 to 4 milligrams per day but only 10 to 40 percent of the zinc we ingest is absorbed. This poses a special problem for people with IBD because zinc is absorbed from the colon, which is likely to have been removed or flushed with chronic diarrhea.

Although zinc is available in all plants and animals, zinc from animal sources, such as meat and fish, is twice as well absorbed by the human body as that from other sources. The zinc found in many plant sources is poorly absorbed because it is bound up with indigestible substances. The best plant sources include beans and whole grains; among meats the best are red meat, oysters, and poultry. Food processing eliminates much zinc along with other minerals and vitamins.

Many Americans cut down on meat to reduce cholesterol, so unless they increase their consumption of whole grains and beans, they won't get enough zinc. As with many other nutrients, anyone in our society who doesn't eat large quantities of nutritious food daily may also have a marginal zinc intake. Children, women, the elderly, and the poor usually fall into this category.

But the zinc picture may even be worse than that. Recent government research indicates that, given typical American food preferences, an intake of 3,400 Calories would be required to obtain the 15 milligrams RDA for zinc. Unless you're a teenage boy or a hard-training athlete, it's unlikely that you could eat anywhere near that many Calories. Athletes may even need more zinc, because it may be lost through sweat.

Another factor that can jeopardize the body's zinc supply is alcohol. So add alcoholics to the list of those likely to be zinc-deficient. This is especially harmful during pregnancy, for the fetus may be deficient in zinc.

The Trouble with Too Much Zinc

Considering the magnitude and scope of zinc's role in the body, it may be prudent to supplement zinc in the diet up to the RDA level. But be sensible. The theory that "if a little is good, more is better" does not apply to zinc. Excess zinc reduces the absorption of copper. At ten times the RDA level, zinc even interferes with the body's cholesterol balance, causing a shift toward the harmful kind of cholesterol that causes heart disease. Sensible supplementation makes sense.

Fluorine: The Cavity Fighter

Fluorine is another trace element with a fine line between not enough and too much. In the 1930s, residents of Arizona, Colorado, and the Texas panhandle were in a panic because their teeth were becoming mottled. Chalky spots appeared on the enamel and later turned an unsightly dark brown. Were they being poisoned?

Abnormally high concentrations of fluorine were found in their drinking water. Although disfiguring, the mottled teeth were not a health threat. In fact, the teeth of children in these areas proved to be more resistant to tooth decay than those of children living in areas where the fluorine content was lower. By the 1940s, scientists had found an ideal level of fluorine that would prevent tooth decay without causing mottled teeth. Fluoridating public drinking water to that level, one part per million, is now a scientifically accepted, safe, economical public health measure.

An adult body contains 2 to 3 grams of fluorine, primarily in bones and teeth. This fluorine needs to be replaced as cells turn over. The government's safe and adequate range of intake for most people is 1.5 to 4.0 milligrams. With fluoridated drinking water, that's about what we consume every day, although aluminum-containing antacids and aluminum in drinking water can interfere with fluorine absorption. Toxicity from fluorine, called fluorosis, occurs only with intakes of 20 milligrams or more daily over long periods of time. This is about eight times the normal intake from food and fluoridated water. Severe tooth and bone deformities are the symptoms of fluorosis.

A more common problem, particularly if you live in an area without fluoridated water, is not enough fluorine. Indisputable scientific evidence has found that fluorine is essential to the stability and strength of bones and teeth even though it is not one of the major structural components. Think of fluorine as being like the rubber taps the shoemaker puts on the heels and toes of your shoes to keep them from wearing down.

Fluorine is especially important for developing strong teeth that will last a lifetime. Therefore, it is crucial early in life. Tooth development begins during the tenth to twelfth week of pregnancy, and some studies have found that supplementing the diet of pregnant women with fluorine at that time produces offspring with virtually cavity-proof teeth. Many prenatal supplements now contain fluorine. Many children who live in areas with unfluoridated drinking water now have fluorine applied directly to their teeth by the dentist.

Fluorine may also be important in old age for treatment and prevention of osteoporosis. It cannot take the place of supplemental calcium or hormonal therapy in keeping bones strong, but it may help stop further erosion of calcium from the bones. Some scientists now suggest that a fluorine deficiency may be one of the causes of osteoporosis.

A rumor circulating some years back that fluorine caused cancer kept some communities from fluoridating their water supply. Although this allegation has no basis and has been refuted by the American Cancer Society and the National Cancer Institute, it continues to send many people to the dentist for their fluorine application.

Chromium: The Beer Mineral

When various cultures around the world learned to make beer, they were supplementing their diets not only with B vitamins, but with chromium. Although the B vitamins may be gone from modern beer, beer drinkers can take heart. Your favorite brew is still a good source of chromium.

Imagine people's surprise back in the chrome-plated 1950s, when two U.S. scientists discovered that the shiny metal adorning bumpers and tail fins was actually required by the human body. At 50 to 20 micrograms, the amount needed is very small, but is vital to assist the hormone insulin in its action, which controls glucose metabolism. Although its exact chemical nature is still under study, chromium's active form is called the glucose tolerance factor (GTF).

The body contains very little chromium—about 6 milligrams total. Our chromium content declines with age. When chromium is deficient, insulin function is impaired, and certain forms of diabetes may result. A slight deficiency that might be tolerated in a younger person is thought to cause some cases of adult-onset diabetes, when combined with the natural losses of old age. But this type of diabetes caused by chromium deficiency is rare; most adult-onset diabetes in North America is the result of overweight.

As in the case of selenium, the amount of chromium in foods depends primarily on the amount in the soil. Processing and refining reduce the chromium content of foods considerably. For example, white flour contains much less than whole wheat flour. But don't rush out to buy a chromium supplement. It seems that the best way to obtain chromium containing the crucial GTF is from beef or pork; other good sources are wheat germ or brewer's yeast. Besides, considering the total absence of chromium-deficiency symptoms in this country, it's apparent that a varied and well-balanced diet provides all we need.

Trace Minerals and IBD

Trace minerals should cause folks with IBD to take notice; they're especially vulnerable. Their vulnerability derives from limited diet, chronic diarrhea, and the likelihood of poor absorption due to the illness or surgical removal of part of the bowel. It's important to make up for these possibilities, because trace minerals are essential to good health.

Seafood, especially shellfish, is an excellent source of all trace minerals. Red meat, especially organ meats, is a close second to shellfish as a source of trace minerals. The white meat of finfish and poultry comes next. In the vegetable kingdom, beans and wheat germ are the best sources. Intake of all these foods is seriously limited from time to time by folks with IBD, and many of them are never eaten.

Trace minerals, especially zinc, iodine, copper, and others I haven't mentioned, like manganese, are poorly absorbed from even healthy bowels. In IBD we can expect absorption to be reduced even more dramatically. If you've lost part of the small intestine, absorption will similarly be reduced by absorptive area.

All this adds to the point I've made before: sensible supplementation. I emphasize the word *sensible* because it implies two important points: not excessive and complete. Many supplements contain lots of some vitamins, such as one or two of the Bs, but have no zinc or copper. From my brief essays on nutrition, you can see that teamwork is essential in nutrition. Teamwork among the trace minerals is an excellent example of that concept.

CHAPTER TWENTY-ONE

Electrolytes:
Sodium + Potassium =
Body Currents

Did you know that your body contains electrically charged particles? That's why your doctor can take an electrocardiogram reading from your body, why brushing your hair on a cold morning can make sparks fly, why touching an exposed wire gives you a shock. I'm not talking about enough electricity to light even a small light bulb; I'm talking about the tiny electrical charge necessary to send nerve impulses to your muscles so you can turn thoughts into actions, or if you touch a hot stove, pull back.

Certain mineral salts, called electrolytes, dissolve in water and separate into their electrically charged particles, called ions. As ions they can conduct an electric current. This makes possible the nerve and muscle reactions, including for example, the heartbeat. Nerves are like the electric wires in our homes. They conduct impulses of electricity to all parts of our body. These impulses make our muscles move and are used to sense the environment. For example, visual images are transferred by nerves to our brain; the image travels along the optic nerve as a series of electrical impulses. Our brain transforms these impulses into a visual image that we see. It all happens instantly.

Sodium and potassium are the two most abundant and important electrolytes in our body. Magnesium and calcium also act as electrolytes, but they're secondary to sodium and potassium, which are found throughout nature. Natural foods, such as apples, meat, grains, and vegetables contain much more potassium than sodium. Sodium is excessively abundant as common table salt, sodium chloride. As we'll see later, this abundance causes some problems.

Fluid Balance

In addition to conducting electrical charges, the electrolytes serve another important function. Each of our bodies' 50 trillion cells is bathed in fluid. The membrane of each cell separates its contents from the fluid. This membrane conducts materials in and out; for example water, oxygen, and other nutrients go in, whereas waste products, such as carbon dioxide and some chemicals, go out. The membrane must also allow important chemical products the cell makes as part of its special function to pass. The balance of the electrolytes inside the cell and in the fluid outside each cell regulates the flow of fluids, especially water, in and out. This regulation is critical to the life and function of the cell. Its importance can't be overstated.

If too much fluid goes into the cell, it will swell and stop functioning. In a serious imbalance, when too much fluid goes in, the cell can burst and die. In contrast, if too much fluid leaves the cell, it will shrivel up like a raisin and stop functioning. Either way, if the fluid balance isn't correct, the cell's function will be seriously impaired, if not completely stopped; the cell can sicken and die. I hope you've got the point: fluid balance is a critical function of the electrolytes.

In the fluids bathing the outside of the cell are sodium

and chloride; while inside are potassium and a little chloride. This balance between potassium inside and sodium outside is critically important to all cell functions. It doesn't matter whether the cell is part of the adrenal glands making the hormone adrenaline, if it's in the optic nerve sending visual signals to the brain, or if it's a cell at the base of the intestinal wall: the cell must have the correct potassium-sodium balance to function properly.

Here's where calcium and magnesium are also involved. There's more calcium and magnesium in the fluid outside the cell than in the fluid inside the cell. This balance is also important and depends to some extent on the potassium-sodium balance inside and outside the cell. The ratio of potassium to sodium is important.

Three: The Magic Ratio

Your body maintains a ratio of about three parts potassium to one part sodium. This potassium-sodium ratio is important and enables each cell to perform its special function. Indeed, the ratio is not unique to humans; it's found throughout the animal kingdom. For example, the ratio is about three in beef, deer, elephant, rabbit, chicken, or aardvark.

Vegetables are different. In the vegetable kingdom the ratio of potassium to sodium is very high. It also varies more than in animals. Table 21.1 contains the potassium-sodium content and ratio of some natural foods. This ratio is called the K factor because "K" is the chemical symbol for potassium. It's also the subject of a book on high blood pressure.

Maintaining The Magic Ratio

Suppose the extracellular fluid, blood, becomes over-supplied with sodium. How would the body return things to normal? There are two ways to deal with the situation in addition to eating correctly.

TABLE 21.1
Potassium Sodium Content of Some Foods
"The Cost of Processing"
Per Serving

Food	Sodium	Potassium	K factor
	(mg)	(mg)	(Potassium: Sodium)
Beef	44	311	7.00
Hot dog (all beef)	461	71	0.15
Chicken breast	80	360	4.50
Fast food or frozen and breaded	1012	360	0.40
Corn (fresh)	11	219	20.00
Corn (canned)	680	219	0.30
Corn flakes	351	26	0.07
Beans	8	456	57.00
Beans (canned)	1161	620	0.53
Broccoli	12	143	11.92
Broccoli with sauce	391	225	0.58
Nabisco Shredded Wheat	6	150	25.00

Excreting sodium is the simplest, most direct way to re-store balance. This is one of the many jobs of the kidneys, the organs that produce urine. If the kidneys don't do this job well, the body responds by raising the blood pressure. Higher blood pressure forces sodium from the kidneys, but high blood pressure is also an illness that should be avoided. As an aside, it's also important to drink enough water for the kidneys to work with.

Another way to reduce the oversupply of sodium is to dilute it. The body does this by simply retaining fluid. Look at it this way. While the K factor is important, each cell is faced with a concentration of sodium in the fluid surround-ing it. Concentration means so much sodium per volume of fluid; if the volume of fluid is increased, the ratio on the basis of volume is reduced. In other words, retain more fluid, dilute the sodium, and make the ratio seem lower. Thus, fluid retention is a device the body uses to reduce the concentration of sodium. In other words, fluid retention is associated with excess sodium. It's also a sign of heart trouble, but that's another subject.

Normally these two mechanisms work together. The blood pressure goes up to excrete excess sodium, while the body retains extra fluid. You notice this when it happens, because your rings, belt, or shoes feel a little tighter. In some people, if this happens often enough, the blood pressure becomes permanently raised. High blood pressure from excessive sodium is the outcome. I've written an entire book on this subject.

Dietary Potassium and Sodium: "We Are What We Eat"

Because the body raises the blood pressure to get rid of excess sodium, scientists began to look at the urine of large populations to see whether there was any agreement with the idea that excessive sodium produces high blood pressure. Their findings were startling. When the K factor in the urine of a population is three or more—that's three potassium to every sodium—only 1 to 2 percent of the people get high blood pressure. If the K factor drops to one, however, meaning there's as much or more sodium than potassium, on average, about 20 to 25 percent of the people will have high blood pressure. It's that clear! Scientists don't even debate it anymore.

From studies like these and others, we know that the best diet contains a K factor of three or more. Intuitively, this seems correct because natural foods contain a K factor of 3 or more and the ratio of 3 found in animal foods, such meat, milk, and eggs, is low compared to vegetable foods, where the ratio is often 10 or more, up to 150. So, a natural foods diet, with no salt added, will contain much more potassium than sodium. By some estimates the dietary K factor of a natural diet could be as high as 8 for people who are moderate meat eaters to a high of 16 for vegetarians. Take a look at Table 21.1 and you'll see that natural foods contain much more potassium than sodium. Man-made foods or processed natural foods are a major departure. In fact, this departure is important to people with bowel problems; especially if they get diarrhea.

Our "Sea of Salt"

Salary, the word that describes our income, is derived from two words: "salt ration." That's correct; salt was once so scarce it was a medium of exchange, like gold dust in 1849 in California, or like money today. Now salt is so plentiful that we use it to melt ice on sidewalks. Unfortunately, we also use too much of it in preparing food.

Table salt is sodium chloride; the same stuff our kidneys work so hard to excrete. Most Americans get from 7 to 10 grams of it daily. That's from 3 to 5 grams of sodium! It doesn't sound like much, but we need a minimum of only 200 milligrams of sodium daily and the government says a safe range is 1,100 to 3,000 milligrams or 1 to 3 grams. Since salt (sodium chloride) is just under 40 percent sodium, 7 to 10 grams of salt is an enormous amount of sodium compared to our requirement. This excess simply obliterates the K factor of three by reducing it to less than one!

Table 21.1 shows you why table salt is not always the culprit. If there's anything we can say about processed food, it's that it's excessive in sodium. Compare, for example, the K-factor ratios of beef to hot dogs, or corn to canned corn and corn flakes. You'll see what I mean when I say we live in a "sea of salt."

Potassium: Sodium Requirement

A 150-pound person's body contains more than 8 ounces of potassium and 3 of sodium. That's a ratio of about three. Because our kidneys are so good at retaining salt, we can get along with 200 milligrams of sodium daily. Our kidneys are even better at conserving chloride, so we can get along with even less of that. The Food and Nutrition Board recommends a safe and adequate range of sodium of from 1,100 to 3,300 milligrams daily. They don't say we require it; they say it's safe and the word *adequate* is redundant.

Potassium, in contrast, is not conserved by the kidneys. There's never been a need, because in more than three million years of human development, sodium and chloride were scarce; however, potassium has always been abundant in natural food. Sodium and chloride were very scarce until the last 150 years, whereas potassium is abundant in natural food and our kidneys release it readily when they produce urine. Therefore, the Food and Nutrition Board places the potassium requirement at from 1,875 milligrams to 5,100 milligrams. That's much higher than sodium. It's very important to everyone; especially people with IBD.

It's unfortunate that the Food and Nutrition Board set the safe and adequate ranges for sodium and potassium before they understood the K factor. Now that we understand the health implications of a K factor of less than three, the numbers should be revised. Although scientific agreement is nearly unanimous, it will be at least five, and probably ten years before the sodium/potassium recommendations are revised. I believe that we should get from 200 to 800 milligrams of sodium and from 2,000 to 4,000 milligrams of potassium daily. The good news is that if you eat a natural diet rich in vegetables, you'll attain these levels without even trying.

Why Not Potassium Supplements?

Potassium supplements should be sold only as prescription drugs because too much potassium taken as supplements can cause serious intestinal problems. Potassium supplements are prescribed when people take medication to control high blood pressure. They're not effective simply to restore balance to a poor diet.

The only solution to inadequate potassium is correct food selection. Table 21.1 will show you that natural foods are fine. Table 21.2 gives some examples of foods that are extra rich in potassium. These foods conveniently provide a potassium boost naturally without problem. In Chapter Three I explained the use of a food diary to make sure they're okay for you.

TABLE 21.2
Convenient Natural Foods Rich in Potassium*
Per Serving

Food	Potassium	K Factor
Avocado	1097	52
Bamboo shoots	640	128
Broad beans	456	57
Kidney beans	713	178
Lima beans	955	238
Peas	644	72
Potato	608	87
Squash	445	445
Apricot	313	313
Banana	451	451
Dried lychee	1110	370
Orange	250	250
Papaya	780	98
Raisins	751	63

*All natural foods have a good K factor, the potassium: sodium ratio. The foods listed here are especially good for potassium. They can be used as "natural" potassium supplements.

IBD: The Dangers of Diarrhea

Electrolytes are important to people with bowel disorders; more important is maintaining a K factor of three or even better. Getting more than 3,000 milligrams of potassium daily is essential. I say this because diarrhea robs the body of potassium. It makes things even worse by causing dehydration. When you get diarrhea, or have watery stools all the time as many people with IBD, two things happen: You lose water continuously (although you can make it up by simply drinking more) and you continuously lose potassium (which you can make up only by eating correctly).

People with inflammatory bowel disorders should strive for a dietary K factor of at least three and preferably five or more to be on the safe side. It's not hard; when we get into the next section we'll review some easy techniques, but I'll say it once again: Eat natural foods, especially vegetables.

Dehydration and Electrolyte Imbalance: "Be on Your Guard"

When you become dehydrated and lose potassium, your body can't function properly. When it happens to athletes, they either lose the race or drop out. But most of us don't function at the outward limit of our ability; we simply get along in the world of work. But don't get the idea it doesn't matter. It matters very much.

Dehydration and electrolyte imbalance show up at first as a lack of energy and fatigue. If it gets worse, dizzy spells, fainting spells, and disorientation result. For most people it never goes beyond the statements: "I feel so tired. I can't get moving," or "I've had this headache and I feel so tired." In my correspondence with folks who have IBD, I noticed that many complain about being "tired" or "lacking energy." While there are many reasons for these feelings, one of them needn't be poor electrolyte balance and chronic borderline dehydration.

If you experience bouts of diarrhea, you've got to be on your guard. Table 21.2 lists foods that are especially rich in potassium. The banana, if fully ripe, is a favorite that can be tolerated by many people with bowel disorders (Chapter Two). Eat plenty of them. And be sure to drink enough water.

Chicken Soup

When you're sick, you may think longingly of chicken soup. Not the canned or dry-mix variety, but the old-fashioned chicken soup that Grandmother used to make. Chicken soup earned its reputation as a miracle drug by helping to relieve the symptoms and speed recovery from colds and flu with their associated stomach upset and diarrhea. The soup works in two ways. Research proved that factors from the chicken fat and protein increased metabolism. This provides a lift. More important, the soup was a treasure of minerals, especially potassium. Also, the vapors, with the aroma and a little garlic, would help to clear nasal congestion. But let's get back to the electrolytes.

When you become dehydrated and lose potassium, you become tired and lack energy. That's why world-class athletes are so concerned about their food intake and electrolyte balance. For them it's the difference between winning and losing. For a person with diarrhea, it's the difference between feeling good and feeling terrible with a certain loss of energy. Old-fashioned chicken soup solved this problem very nicely. Made from the bones and some meat from the chicken, old-fashioned chicken soup was rich in potassium and low in sodium. It also contained some magnesium, the unsung mineral I talk about so much. The mere act of drinking chicken soup restored fluid. The result: electrolyte balance was restored, cells were rehydrated, and you feel well again.

Alas, I must finish this section with a word of caution. Most modern, prepackaged or canned soups are an electrolyte disaster! That's right. They contain an excess of sodium and very little potassium. In fact, some dry soup mixes are more than 20 percent salt! That's not what we're after and it's why I emphasize chicken soup made the old-fashioned way.

PART THREE

Human

Considerations

Nutrition and diet are actually about people and society, although we often separate food from nutrition. This separation is complete and routine with TPN and almost complete with nutritional products like Criticare HN and Vital HN (see Chapter Eight); the separation happens to a lesser extent with vitamin and mineral supplements. Even though products like Criticare and Vital aren't really food, people who need them either accept them as is or complain about taste, texture, and wanting to "sink their teeth into real food." These Enteral products aren't designed with taste appeal as a primary consideration, but it proves that the human factor is important whenever food is involved.

Stress and emotion have much to do with the way we process food. Is Eileen correct when she says, "Stress causes flare-ups and foods only aggravate them"? If so, we must examine the issues surrounding food and stress and try to bring one or both into a common focus. Certainly our emotions influence the food we eat. Conversely, the food we eat influences our emotions. So if stress, emotions, or food causes IBD flare-ups, how do you separate one from the other?

Exercise is a strange topic to discuss in a book about diet and IBD. As a biochemist and a nutritionist, I know that exercise can work wonders and that it has a strong effect on our eating habits. It reduces stress, helps to normalize metabolism, and makes people feel better. They feel better about themselves psychologically and they feel better physically. If there's any problem with exercise, it's the mistaken notion that exercise has to cause pain and make you tired.

I want to express my thoughts on how a chronic illness like IBD gets started, why these illnesses seem to be increasing, and what might happen if we don't take some research efforts more seriously. Then I'd like to propose some thought for a new effort in the support group concept—an idea to help people get more involved in self-health management.

Anecdotal Information

Anecdotal information is generally scoffed at by scientists, but it's used all the time in medicine. For example, a doctor will typically watch one patient to see if a plan works for this person; if it does, the doctor will try it again, and if the results continue to be positive, it becomes the office routine. By trial and error, some anecdotal observations stand the test of time and evolve into science. They're usually small things that wouldn't be the subject of major research. I once gave a talk on arthritis and poked fun at copper bracelets, only to read later that one researcher decided that anything in such widespread use should be tested, and he proved it worked to a modest extent. It also put into perspective some other observations involving copper. I was amazed at how quickly scientists could explain "why" it worked. I wondered where they had been hiding. But didn't sayings like "every child needs the January sun" and "an apple a day," or putting nails in apples start as folkways that at first seemed foolish? If they may do some good and are not harmful, why not follow them cautiously?

I've collected anecdotal reports from folks with IBD. Some of them use supplements to an extreme. They claim the supplements help them; as a group they seem more cheerful, positive about the future, and in control. Some claim that it saved them from surgery. I simply don't know. I do know that good nutrition, a positive outlook, and good condition go together. I've seen it in research studies and have heard too many people tell me that nutrition makes a big difference to ignore them. Although we don't know what causes IBD, we do know that good nutrition with a few commonsense precautions helps. So why not give them a try? They can't do any harm and have the potential to do much good.

CHAPTER TWENTY-TWO

Stress: An
Overworked Word

Have you ever heard of an international track record being set in an empty stadium with one runner and only officials present? Of course not! Track records are set in the stress of competition. Sometimes the second-place runner is so close that a photoelectric timer is necessary to tell who really won. Physiological stress, with a realistic goal, managed by good coaching, fair rules, and honest officials, allows the best to surface.

In contrast, how many times have we heard of someone who cracked under "stress," a child who couldn't live up to his parents' expectations, an executive who had excellent qualifications, but became reclusive and finally had a nervous collapse under the stress of an office environment, or of someone who gets sick and goes from one doctor to another searching for the "cure" for a series of undefined symptoms?

Stress is an overworked word. In the preceding examples, the difference is stress management. Athletes use stress and coaches manage it; they make it work for them. In the everyday environment it's seldom managed; indeed, it's sort of "free-floating." When stress is free-floating, we're left to our own devices. We too often stop trying to thrive and settle for mere survival. And too often the "free-floating" stress in our lives surfaces in the form of illness.

Let me explain what I mean by "free-floating" stress. A friend asked me why the independent, part-time distributors of his products weren't doing better. His sales were actually declining. He put it this way, "Jim, who is our competition?" He went on to tell me how superior his products were to those of his perceived competitors. My answer was simple: "Tom, your only competition is time." I went on to explain that the sociologists have calculated that in the past five years the average person has lost eight hours of discretionary time each week. We've lost it to increases in TV programs, junk mail, fax machines, commuting time, and organizations. I concluded by saying, "Tom, you're competing for people's discretionary time against things you and they can't see. It's like trying to nail a block of gelatin to a tree in June."

Tom's stress is from "free-floating" hassles he can't see. How do you compete with junk mail, TV programs, or long commutes? But that's what he had to do. His solution is clear; if he wants his distributors to be more effective, he's got to teach time management. They have to eliminate enough inessential claims on their time to be more productive.

When we can define sources of stress, we can manage ourselves so external hassles don't become internal stress. Then we're in control; we can either neutralize the stress and ignore it, or we can use it to our advantage. But first we must identify the major sources of stress.

Stress and IBD

IBD is not an emotional, psychosomatic illness; that much has been investigated and determined by excellent scientists.

That doesn't mean that IBD flare-ups aren't triggered by stress, however, nor does it mean the IBD doesn't start during a period of unmanageable stress or serious emotional upset. I have found only one or two people with IBD who haven't listed stress as a trigger of flare-ups; instead, they listed the vague symptoms of "fatigue" and "being tired." Let's look at some of the nonfood causes of flare-ups, experienced by a wide cross-section of people.

Nonfood Causes of IBD Flare-ups

This is a sampling of what people said:

ESTHER: Exercise, shopping, lifting children, and keeping up with household demands.

FRED: Seasonal changes, especially spring and fall.

TODD: Withheld emotions; specifically anger, sadness, and resentment. Also overwork.

SHAWN: Lack of sleep.

ANOLA: Occasionally, charcoal lighter fluid when we use it to start a fire on a grill.

IRENE: Family problems and my sinuses. I don't think I breathe right and it makes me nervous. Then the nerves trigger an attack.

NILA, BECKY, CAROLE, HANNA, AND OTHERS: Anytime I get really upset or exercise too much. Hard housecleaning will do it. Anytime I get really excited about something. It started with my wedding.

L. R.: Not getting enough sleep due to major problems either in the family or at work.

PATRICIA: I can relate my first attack directly to the death of my mother. Each flare-up relates to some stressful event.

MARY SUE: When responsibilities mount up and things I can't change get out of control. I feel insecure and the attack happens.

LEWIS, A DENTIST: Physical fatigue. Too much time on my feet and working on patients.

MARC: I'm a professional internalizer. This has not helped marital harmony and my flare-ups are directly attributed to this.

JANET: Not enough sleep. I recently quit my job and started working part-time so I could get more sleep. It helped.

DIANE: Getting chilled, especially along with lack of rest.

ROBERT: Although my doctor says stress is not a cause, my experience says otherwise.

JANET: My husband causes flare-ups!

RICHARD: Cold, damp weather causes flare-ups for me. In fact, I can get it from going into an air-conditioned store on a hot summer day.

GAIL: Travel. In my previous job I had to travel with little notice. I would get fatigue, jet lag, and a flare-up of my Crohn's. I changed jobs!

ANNETTE: I've been verbally abused all my life. I married an alcoholic and took verbal abuse for eighteen years until he quit drinking. I just completed an R.N. degree at age 41. No one can tell me stress isn't involved!

MRS. ARTHUR O: Spring always brings attacks. I recover by fall but then I often get a kidney stone.

ROBERT: Sudden changes in my routine that I can't control will bring on a flare-up.

What Can We Learn from This?

Stress counts! So do other things that relate to stress or create it, such as fatigue, sensitivities, and overwork. Stress and fatigue go together. This doesn't mean that I believe stress causes IBD or that IBD is psychosomatic, only that stress can bring on the flare-up. Is there any other illness that helps us to see this more clearly? Let's consider adult acne.

Adult Acne

Some people start getting acne as adults, say in their mid-twenties, even though their skin was clear all their lives, especially as teenagers. One doctor says, "I think some people are destined to get acne and it comes out later in them; they can't escape it." Along with that speech he prescribes the standard antibiotic and the acne clears in about six months; if it's a woman, she sometimes gets a yeast infection as a side effect of the antibiotic, but research shows there's more involved.

Other doctors do more serious analysis and they find that stress acts as a trigger in many of these people. They also noticed that acne is a side effect of a well-known high blood pressure medication. "What do they both have in common?" they asked. "Changes in hormone balance" was the answer. Stress decreases the level of the male hormone testosterone, as do some medications. Since we all have both male and female hormones in our blood, the hormone balance is essential and is upset by stress and some medications.

The Acne Lesson

My objective in telling you this about acne is not to pretend that changes in hormone balance cause IBD to flare up. That might be true, but it'll take a very large and sophisticated research project to find out. My objective is to point out that stress influences the very chemicals that regulate our bodily functions and shows itself in ways even experts don't always expect. Therefore, the fact that stress is related to flare-ups doesn't mean that it's a cause-and-effect relationship.

Stress also influences our immune response. It doesn't increase its potential; it decreases it. The stress can come from such things as emotions, fatigue, a chemical, or a chill. Studies on Olympic skiers proved quite clearly that if they got chilled, they were much more likely to get colds and the flu than if they weren't. Reread Diane's and Richard's comments.

Sound familiar? Reread the anecdotal reports I described and see if fatigue, chills, and other forms of stress aren't listed as triggers of a flare-up. If IBD is similar to autoimmune diseases like rheumatoid arthritis, it all fits a very nice pattern with one important lesson: You've got to learn to identify and manage your stressors! But first, let's talk about chemical sensitivities.

Chemical Sensitivities

In Chapter Six I listed beets as a cause of flare-ups. I heard that from many people. As one woman, Mrs. Arthur O, put it: "Eating a beet, even if it's cooked and peeled, will just about kill me!" Other people were content with simply listing beets as a food that causes flare-ups. But what about the comments made by other people: Anola and lighter fluid, Fred and seasonal changes, and Irene and her sinuses? These are all sensitivities. We can take a lesson here from arthritis and asthma.

Arthritis and Asthma

When I wrote *The Arthritis Relief Diet*, I urged people to keep a diary to identify things that caused flare-ups. I received this letter from one woman.

> *Dear Dr. Scala:*
> *I was so delighted. My arthritis flared up so bad I was bedridden for two days. I had been to a cocktail party and ate some chicken liver hors d'oeuvres. The next morning I couldn't get out of bed.*
> *I'm happy because I had forgotten just how far I had come. My diary taught me that chicken liver was a clear trigger for my flare-ups and I forgot it. I'll never do that again.*
>
> > *Sincerely,*
> > *Helen*

Helen's letter is clear. Something in those livers triggers a flare-up. I don't know what it is, nor does she, nor does her doctor—and we don't need to know. Helen must simply *avoid chicken livers!* Her life will be just as satisfying without them.

Asthma is similar in its effects. Pat and her husband moor their boat near ours. Pat only needs to be near fresh marine varnish to experience an asthma attack. If she doesn't leave quickly, she requires medication. Pat has a sensitivity to something in fresh marine varnish that comes out in the fumes. She's got to avoid fresh varnish; it's that simple.

Pat and Irene have sensitivities. So do Anola, Fred, and many others. How else do you explain lighter fluid, seasonal response, and sinuses? Something in the air causes a sensitivity to emerge and the flare-up gets started. In rheumatoid arthritis, flare-ups result from changes in the barometric pressure, as happens when a cold front passes through. Some scientists actually proved it by putting arthritic volunteers in a phytotron, a large chamber for growing plants in which changes in pressure and weather can be simulated. In England, the early fall is called the arthritis season. It's the time of frequent weather changes and lots of arthritic flare-ups; now we know why.

Finding the Stress Points

It's interesting to talk about the links between stress, sensitivity, and fatigue, but it's more helpful to identify the source, then deal with it. The best way I know to identify things that cause a flare-up is to keep the food diary described in Chapter Three. All you've got to do is keep track of what you eat and drink and note anything that's different or unusual. A couple of lines is sufficient. You'll soon discover what causes your flare-ups. Then you can deal with them more effectively. Sensitivities should be part of your vocabulary by now, so let's deal with them first.

Sensitivities

Notice I use the word *sensitivity*, not *allergy*. That's because people seem to be "sensitive" to things, but not allergic to them. Read what Anola said; she's *sensitive* to the presence of charcoal lighter fluid. There's something in it that she's sensitive to. How do you deal with these things?

You avoid them, that's how! Think of the most severe sensitivity; an alcoholic and alcohol. There's only one thing an alcoholic can do to remain sober: stay away from alcohol. Sensitivities are more difficult to deal with than allergies because they aren't as clearly identified and they require a different type of willpower. But they're just as important. I realize that alcoholism is a hereditary, treatable disease, and I know that alcoholics are missing an enzyme and the blood alcohol-brain barrier is sensitized. The increased sensitivity to alcohol leads to dependency, and the only solution is to stay away from it. Similarly, Anola should not get near lighter fluid!

Fatigue

Fatigue and chronic illness are like oil and water; they don't mix! Fatigue favors stress; in fact, fatigue and stress aren't an additive effect, they're synergistic, meaning that putting the two of them together has a greater effect than if you simply added the effect of each together. It's as if one plus one totals five. And avoiding fatigue doesn't always mean getting more rest.

Fighting Fatigue

Answer a few questions. How much sleep do you get? If you're an adult and you're getting from six to eight hours nightly, fatigue is not from lack of sleep. Experts say that fewer than six hours of sleep regularly is not enough for most people and that more than eight hours is unnecessary and will make you feel tired! Sleeping between six and eight hours each night is adequate; the details are mostly habit. If you're not in that sleep range, try changing something to get there. If you can't, you should discuss it with a doctor.

Second question: Is your nutritional status as good as it should be? One question I'm always asked when I try to motivate people to take nutrition seriously is, "Dr. Scala, how will I know better nutrition is having an effect?" I've learned that people want to see results quickly, so I tell them that within three weeks they'll sleep more soundly and wake up more easily. They'll also have more energy and stamina. There are other signals, such as improved fingernail quality, but the ability to sleep and awaken from sleep feeling good are two very obvious improvements.

Though stimulants, like coffee, are not heavily used by the people who shared information with me, they are a major cause of fatigue. Stimulants pick you up and keep you alert, but when you "come down," you're more tired due to the reverse effect. Caffeine is an addictive drug. Therefore, if you drink coffee, tea, or caffeinated soft drinks, reduce your consumption to the equivalent of only one or two cups daily. These beverages could be making you feel tired even when you aren't.

If you aren't using supplements as I discussed in chapters Seven and Eight, you're depriving yourself of certain nutrients. With a chronic illness like IBD, you can't possibly be getting everything from your food. In fact, I'd double the plan I outlined in chapters Seven and Eight and take the full RDA of all vitamins and minerals! I'd even take an extra RDA of the B complex of vitamins and vitamin C.

How's your carbohydrate consumption? Is it mostly in the form of complex carbohydrates as I discussed in Chapter Thirteen, or is it in simple sugar? One study showed that people with IBD ate more sugar than average. If your carbohydrate intake comes from sugar, shift to complex-carbohydrate and high-fiber foods. The stress of large swings in blood sugar, due to ingesting too much sugar, produces fatigue and causes anxiety; together, that's stress.

Next question: Do you get some exercise every day? I don't mean running from responsibility nor a daily 3-mile jog. It's fine if you can jog 3 miles, but it's unnecessary for most folks, especially if they've got IBD. What I'm looking for is a nice walk, short swim, bike ride, or some other moderate activity that gets the vital fluids moving. Soft and easy low-impact aerobic exercise is an excellent way to start. I've discussed the value of exercise in Chapter Twenty-three.

You might think, "I'm worried about fatigue and he's talking about exercise. What's going on here?" It's really very simple. Fatigue is characterized by an accumulation of waste chemicals in our tissues; exercise increases our metabolism and helps to get rid of them. That's why people who exercise have a reduced risk of cancer. But why aren't people who exercise as tired? Because while you're doing moderate exercise, such as walking, your metabolism increases by about 20 percent; that's more than enough to do the job. Exercising provides a physiological and psychological lift and actually gives you more energy. And, you can smell the roses on the walk.

One more question: Are you confusing fatigue with boredom? The solution for boredom is goal setting and making better use of your time. In the Suggested Reading section I've listed a good book on stress and a tape on goal setting. If you apply the book on stress by Dr. Hanson, and the tape on goal setting by Dr. Viscott, boredom will disappear for good. In our fast-moving world, no one should be bored.

Externalizing

A friend of mine, Mary Ann Baker of Tucson, conducts a weight-loss program and uses the concept of the "Fat Bag." It goes like this:

Everyone who enters Mary Ann's group makes a plain canvas bag. Each week when they meet, Mary Ann provides a large container of sand and two scales—a large one for the dieters and a small one for the canvas fat bags. Every time a person loses a pound of weight, they put a pound of sand in their fat bag. If they backslide and gain back a pound, it comes out of the bag! At 10 pounds they get another bag of a different color and the retired bag goes to their trophy case. Some of Mary Ann's graduates have 15 full bags in a trophy case. That's 150 pounds of lost fat!

Some of the people who don't have trophy cases to display their progress used a fireplace mantel or some other shelf. It's a way of externalizing goals. Making the first bag represents and quantifies the first goal; each week there's an opportunity to put some sand in it. Then, when it's full, the second bag is started and the next goal is quantified and externalized. Another good aspect of Mary Ann's method is the group support that accompanies the visual goal. It works.

Every goal that's worth pursuing can be quantified and externalized.

Neutralizing Stress

"God, give me the serenity to accept the things I cannot change, the ability to change the things I can, and the wisdom to know the difference."

That's the Serenity Prayer for children and friends of alcoholics. It summarizes what we can do about stress. If we study it, we recognize that stress is an inner conflict, not some outside force that can't be seen.

Most of my correspondents listed stress as a cause of flare-ups. Of 60 people who responded in detail at one meeting, only 5 didn't list stress, but they did identify fatigue. Of those who mentioned stress and elaborated, about 50 percent identified external sources of stress; for example, Janet clearly identified her husband. But Marc is the most honest of all when he labels himself a "professional internalizer." Lots of people say the same thing. The stress is within us. We can identify three solutions for Janet, such as: dump the husband; go to a marriage counselor; or apply the Serenity Prayer. The first may not be a viable solution; the second might improve the marriage if the husband gets involved, but the third solution is the only one she can control. There's one thing Janet can change—herself. She's got the desire and the capability because she's completely in charge of herself, and avoiding Crohn's flare-ups is enough motivation.

Now I'd like to focus on Marc's personal assessment: being a "professional internalizer." How do you stop being a professional internalizer? By externalizing your problems; that's how. The first step is to start talking about the source with someone who will help you find a solution. Start with your IBD support group. The folks there can empathize with your illness and the effect stress has on your life.

People to People

Your support group already has the foundation for group discussions. Start with them. Then find a speaker or a guest expert who understands the Alanon approach. This approach was developed by those in one of the most stressful of all environmental situations: being the child, spouse, or close friend of an alcoholic or drug addict. These techniques and methods are designed to help you deal with the stress caused by your environment. It helps you learn to "change the things you can." You get to know yourself and understand why you let things beyond your control bother you.

You *can* change how you deal with your external environment so it doesn't become a source of internal stress. The emphasis is on you! What is stressful to you might be a pleasantly competitive environment for someone else. It's all in the eye of the beholder. Other people have had the same problems you have—only worse. You can learn from them and the experts. All you need is the group.

If you're not a member of the National Foundation for Ileitis and Colitis, join. Get to your local support group and raise the issue of dealing with stress, anxiety, and emotional issues. Get a group started. If there's no money for a speaker, or an expert isn't willing to speak *gratis*, invite someone from Alanon. Have them explain how their program works. You'll be amazed how easily it can be applied to your needs.

Stress Is Within: Dump It

Stress is within us. It evolves from many things. With Hanna it was the wedding; with Marc it's internalizing external problems. It can also be physical; for some it's getting cold, for others it's excess weight. Everyone who has IBD is under the stress of a chronic illness and the side effects of medication. There's no single thing that can be called stress. But each thing that leads to stress must be dealt with by goal setting. That's what we've got to deal with next.

First, you've got to distinguish controllable from noncontrollable hassles. A typical controllable hassle is a pet. My family participated in a psychological study to identify hassles. Surprisingly, the study, which included many families, disclosed that pets are a big hassle. So why have them? If you have one and it's a hassle, recognize that you chose the hassle. And learn how to change your behavior to accommodate the pet. Or, don't complain about excess stress that results from having the pet.

A typical noncontrollable hassle might be the public transportation system you've got to use. You're trapped into using it, so don't waste time complaining. If you've got to do something, find the time to organize an action group to demand improvements. If you don't want to do that, don't let it get to you; instead, learn to laugh at it. Also, learn to cope and make it constructive. For example, leave a half hour early with the objective of using the time for something constructive. I know a person who did it by purchasing a Walkman and listening to tapes of good books. He's the most well-read nonreader I know.

Set Goals

Setting goals is difficult. At some point goals must be so realistic they can be included in daily activities. Reread the "Fat Bag" technique. It has made a realistic goal, the loss of 10 pounds (or 5 pounds), external, so you can hold it in your hand. When they aren't realistic, unachieved goals create more stress for the goal-setter. Let's explore two simple goals for people with IBD.

Goal 1: Food Diary

On the surface, keeping a food diary sounds easy. You already do it intuitively, but should do it consistently on a daily basis. First, decide what constitutes a flare-up. For some folks it may be an experience with pain too difficult to describe; for others, it's a bad bout with diarrhea. Quantify it for yourself and then identify things that cause it to happen.

A food diary is essential to keep track of what, when, where, and how you eat. Then, identify how you feel. Is anything unusual? Has anything improved? Once you've identified a flare-up food, what do you plan to do about it? That's one goal; you'll probably want to put it out of your life forever. Suppose you're invited to someone's house for dinner; do you share your list of things you can't eat? You should. These are all part of goal-setting, but in that case it's a short-term goal of not offending someone because you're watching your food intake.

Goal 2: Stool Consistency

There's been sufficient research that proves stool consistency can be controlled by food, specifically by intake of dietary fiber. Whether you've got a pouch, colostomy, or have had no surgery, it's something you should control. Most people I've talked with already do so intuitively with fiber, calcium, iron and calcium, clay, and other things, including prescription drugs. Why not take control of your life and set the goal?

I'm not recommending that you go from numerous watery bowel movements every day to one nice consistent movement. Instead, I'm proposing you set a goal to get as much control as possible with food, supplemental fiber, and by medication. Don't settle for anything less than the perfection of control.

How will you work with your doctor on this one? Do you need to? Is it something you should get your support group working on? Some will say yes and others no. Think it through and make it part of your day-to-day activities.

Sources of Help

Most people never set goals, so the experts focus their efforts on helping regular folks with the everyday objectives of life. These include work, family needs, leisure-time activities, and other things that bring personal fulfillment. However, don't let the fact that you must focus on cutting stress or beefing up your fiber intake deter you. The techniques apply to everything and they work.

Externalize: Goal Board

The most effective way to externalize goals is to write them on 3 by 5 cards and put them on a goal board. My goal board is 2 feet by 3 feet. I devote 15 minutes a day to it. Across the top are about five 3 by 5 note cards containing my most important goals. I work down and across to the sub-goals necessary to achieve those goals. Each one features a date and clear concise statements. Books have been written on the subject, but I believe the tape by Dr. Viscott is the best. You can listen to it often; each time you do you'll hear a new approach or find a new meaning in something he says.

Portability

Goals clearly conceived fit neatly on 3 by 5 note cards. Make a duplicate set of the three most important goals and carry them with you every day. When there's a free moment or two, look at one of them and think about what it says. The advantage of the 3 by 5 card approach is that you can get short-term and intermediate goals that are part of a larger long-term goal. This is like having a 1-pound fat bag that you carry to work each day to keep you honest while you're on a diet. Before long you'll start to visualize yourself achieving it. That's an important step.

Visualization

I had the privilege of hearing a lecture given by the famous sculptor Ivan Boedervsky. Most questions following the lecture involved specific works he had done; then he pointed to the raised hand of a young boy in the audience.

The question was simple: "How do you know what to make from a piece of rock?"

Ivan answered very quickly: "God placed the work in the rock and all I do is chip away the excess." There was some hushed snickering from many adults, and Boedervsky put his hand up to quiet them. "I visualize the work and then take away the excess stone, but the work is in the rock. Sometimes it takes me a long time to see it, but when I do it's just a matter of work." He was serious. I believe he's made a statement we can all learn from. He said to visualize.

Once you visualize what you want to become, once you can see yourself doing it or living it, you will achieve it. And this can apply to your health. Let me put it in the words of Hanna who said it so well:

> X rays showed the disease was spread throughout my intestines; they said the best they could do was to remove the worst parts. Since it wasn't an emergency, I convinced them to wait for a few months while I psyched myself up for the surgery. I'd lie in the bed and see myself well, picturing the disease localizing to a point that it could all be removed. It was much later that I learned visualization techniques that I realized I had been using it! I can still see my doctor's beaming face when I awoke and he said "Hanna, we got it all!" It was localized in just three places!

Did Hanna's mental preparation help her achieve the goal she sought? Was it realistic of her to "psych" herself up for the surgery? I ask anyone who reads this: why not?

We become what we visualize for ourselves!

Positive Thinking

Mental conditioning can be practiced all day every day. This is in contrast to physical conditioning, which requires activity, special equipment, time, and other restrictions. Mental conditioning requires much more self-discipline, however. Positive thinking, positive mental attitude, positive recognition, and positive action without reward are necessary. Let's explore how each of these helps.

You must first apply the maxim that something positive exists in every situation. Find the positive and build on it; don't dwell on the negative. One woman, Nancy, gave me a beautiful example:

Her son came home from school with three "Ds," one "F," and a "C." She was heartbroken; here was her pride and joy on his way to nowhere, never achieving what she and his father had hoped for him. But she's a positive woman and didn't want him to be depressed, so she thought a moment and said, "Jack, I'm so proud you're my son!" He was astonished and said sheepishly, "Why? I thought you'd be angry." Nancy replied clearly, "I'm proud that I have a son who doesn't cheat."

The ability to see the positive in such a poor report card is truly positive thinking. Nancy is about the best example I know of a person whose thought process automatically responds to everything in a positive manner. With Nancy, a positive outlook is automatic and contagious, but it's the result of positive self-discipline throughout her life. Her son, Jack, went on to become one of the world's best motivational speakers!

Positive Mental Attitude

A positive mental attitude is a little more subtle. It requires searching for the silver lining in the cloud that's on the horizon. It's the attitude that the future is always a little brighter than the present. It's the attitude that allows people to see beyond the years and plan for a brighter future.

The Roman philosopher Cicero wrote of people planting olive orchards, recognizing that they would derive little benefit from them in their lifetime. He observed that they would be there to feed future generations. That is a positive mental attitude—the ability to strive constantly for a better future.

A second excellent example is my mother. I found a bag of dried peach pits in her study. When I offered to throw them out, her reply was immediate: "Oh no, Jimmy, I often substitute for the fourth grade and I use them to have the children make turkeys." She went on to explain how she uses toothpicks, glue, cotton, and some paper to make miniature turkeys with third and fourth grade students around Thanksgiving. You think, so what? Well, at the time my mother was 76 years old! She was still planning how she would keep students productively occupied as a substitute teacher. That fall she was often asked to substitute and she used those peach pits! And now, at age 83, she still does the same thing. Now that's a positive mental attitude!

Positive Recognition

Positive recognition is the easiest of all. You only have to say something nice to someone. Suppose it's a waitress. Before you order say, "What a nice smile you've got," or "That color is very becoming," or "Your walk sure has a bounce to it." The idea is simple: Find some way to recognize something good in your fellow humans. This recognition will come back to you many times over and you'll start to find good things in yourself. If you learn to find and call attention to something good in others, it will become second nature to you and fertilize your new positive thoughts and attitudes.

Mental Conditioning: Positive Action

Last is action. You need to love yourself, and there's no better way than doing something positive anonymously. Help a stranger, give an anonymous gift, send a note to someone, and sign it, "an admirer." But, also do it so people know you do it. If someone does something well, give them a "thumbs-up" sign. It's a short note from you to them with something positive for them, such as, "Dear Kim, I sure enjoyed the way you played that piece on the piano yesterday. It showed excellent progress on your part. Love, Dad." Try it with an employee, a friend, a boss, a colleague—anyone.

Sound corny? Don't kid yourself. Think of how you'd feel

if you got one! If you start now, you'll be surprised how effectively these actions will condition your positive mental processes. You'll need it because you've got an illness that won't quit, fueled by stress that won't quit. The only way to beat stress is to work to maintain mental conditioning as much as a world-class athlete works to maintain physical conditioning.

Simplify

Goal setting does one more thing that most of us fail to do. Simplify! Reread the comment by Annette. She's lived a dysfunctional family life and she's also gone to school at night to become an R.N. That's a complicated life. She has a right to say she's under stress. But there's a solution for both verbal abuse and living with an alcoholic; it's called Alanon.

Alanon makes a major contribution to improving life in a dysfunctional family like Annette's. It has a 12-Step program that works. This is goal setting done for you by someone else. The "steps" are 12 clear goals and you're told to finish one step before you start the next. It works one step at a time. It worked for Annette. Becoming an R.N. is another important step for her. She's now independent! No need to depend on someone else; there's always a job for her if she needs to go out on her own. That's the power of setting goals.

CHAPTER TWENTY-THREE

Exercise:
The Best Medicine

As an aviation cadet in the Air Force I was faced with an important afternoon check ride with an Air Force instructor known for his willingness to flunk cadets. I was apprehensive and decided to spend the morning studying. But trying to study was impossible. I was so tense and nervous I was like a coiled spring. I then recalled an article written by Chuck Yeager before he became famous. In the article he said that when he had a tough flight he would run a few miles to relax.

I put the books away and instead of running, I swam about a half mile. Then I ate a light lunch with my squadron and went for the check flight. It was the best flight I ever had. In thinking over the flight, I realized that I was completely relaxed; I was in control of myself.

What Does Exercise Do?

Exercise and a good diet are synergistic—the sum is greater than its parts. Simply put, if you add the benefits of exercise to a good diet, you get something even better than you might expect. Whenever you increase your activity, you notice your heart beating faster, which is a major objective of exercise. Think of it as a diet dealing with the most important of all the nutrients—oxygen. We can go without food, vitamins, and minerals for months; we can go without water for days, but we can go without oxygen for only a few minutes at most. It's that important.

Oxygen, like all nutrients, is delivered to the tissues by the blood. When we increase our blood flow, we deliver nourishing oxygen more rapidly and efficiently to every tissue. It also removes waste materials from the tissues. As our muscle tone improves from exercise, more blood capillaries develop and the entire process becomes more efficient. (Unfortunately, the converse of that is also true: if we don't exercise, we lose that efficiency.) More important, exercise delivers oxygen and other nutrients to the tissues where the movement is taking place, because that is the location of the most active metabolism. It follows that if we flex and move our joints, it will increase the blood flow to them and the surrounding tissues.

Increased blood flow also delivers more oxygen to the brain. This helps us to be more alert, overcome stress, reduce levels of anxiety and depression, and develop a more positive outlook. In fact, research has indicated that exercise helps the body to produce materials that biochemists call the endorphins, which act as natural mood elevators. In short, exercise done regularly has a positive effect both mentally and physically.

Appearance

Muscles are directly involved in exercise and get the most benefit from it; they increase in strength and general tone, which increases their reserve capacity by helping them to become larger. Experts say that exercise builds lean body mass. Muscle is lean tissue; it contains very little fat.

Muscles are generally smooth in appearance. Consequently, as your muscle mass increases, appearance generally improves; lumpy fat disappears. Daily tasks will become easier as your reserve capacity increases. You are kin to the athlete who trains for an event by practicing beyond the demands of the event.

Thriving Verses Surviving: Benefits of More Muscle

If the appearance of increased muscle mass isn't incentive enough, the physical advantage gained in movement and feeling is even better. But you'll never feel the most important advantages—increased basal metabolic rate. We discussed basal metabolism in Chapter Ten; it's the energy your body spends to keep things running. For example, even while you sleep, your heart is beating, your lungs are extracting oxygen from the air, your kidneys are constantly removing wastes from your blood, and your brain is sifting and cataloging the day's information; each organ is active. There's a lot going on. In Chapter Ten we said that basal metabolism accounts for the majority of calories we burn each 24-hour day.

Fat Is Dormant

Since fat is a "dormant" tissue, it uses an absolute minimum of the body's energy. After all, fat is storage energy and God made it for times of scarcity, so it requires only minuscule energy for its maintenance in times of plenty. That's why a fat body has a much lower metabolic rate than a lean body. It's like money in the bank.

Another thing to consider is that much human fat is located just beneath the skin, where it serves as a layer of insulation. This insulating layer of fat keeps body heat in and conserves the energy required to maintain body temperature. This fatty layer of insulation helps to reduce the basal metabolic rate in fat people. In contrast to fat, lean muscle is anything but dormant. Muscle is packed with blood capillaries and even stores its own energy as glycogen. (Glycogen is "animal" starch, which I discussed in Chapter Thirteen.) You might say that God recognized that muscles would need quick energy and couldn't bother with mobilizing fat reserves in times of need.

Unexpected Benefits

Satisfaction comes with accomplishment; we humans respond to positive reinforcement. You will begin to find satisfaction as you gain flexibility, shift fat to muscle, and can perform tasks you had once thought hopeless. But that's no different than doing anything well.

Mental alertness will improve because improved muscle tone brings improved circulation. It follows that improved circulation brings more oxygen and nourishment to your master organ—the brain.

Sleep will be sounder but not because you are tired; on the contrary, you will have more energy. You sleep better because everything about your body is more efficient. Even though the restorative power of sound sleep remains a scientific mystery, no one can deny its miraculous value, both mental and physical. Sound sleep produces better health.

Bowel function will improve. It's another of the synergistic benefits of exercise with your dietary commitment. The regularity of exercise tones all muscles, including those of the bowel, and helps them to respond easily and regularly.

Bone strength will also increase. A national epidemic of osteoporosis—a decline in bone density due in large part to inadequate dietary calcium and exercise in the childhood and adolescent years—is sweeping the United States. Once women are past the menopause, hormonal changes bring about an acceleration of bone loss, so that bone strength is even more critical. Two factors in osteoporosis require personal control: dietary calcium and exercise. Food and supplements will take care of the calcium, but only you can take care of the exercise!

Never Too Old

Dr. Anthony Albanese conducted a study on postmenopausal women at the Burke Rehabilitation Center. He supplemented their diets with calcium and had them engage in a very modest exercise program, such as walking. In every case the women showed a significant increase in bone density. More important, their energy increased, they felt better, and they became more active. None of this would be either surprising or even important if the women didn't average 82 years in age! They proved that no one is ever too old to improve.

My mother is an excellent example of the ultimate objective of exercise. As I write this she is 83 years old. She spends from 20 to 30 minutes daily on an exercise bicycle in her home. Since she still teaches part-time, I believe exercise has had a positive effect on her. I use my mother to illustrate the point that you are never too old. I expect the same effort from her great-grandchildren, who should be able to fast jog about three miles. This level of activity will lead to all those health benefits I described in the beginning of this chapter. But most important are the mental benefits.

Aerobics

An aerobics craze is sweeping our nation and it's the best thing that could have happened. Some aerobic instructors even conduct classes for people with restricted capabilities. If there's an aerobic class in your community, see if there's a group you can join. Sometimes if you have a group of interested friends, an instructor will hold a special session.

Vigorous Walking

Walking is an excellent exercise. It should be done in comfortable shoes, uninterrupted, with good surroundings, and in safe areas. Most important, it should be done for 30 to 40 minutes at each session. If you can walk twice daily, that's great!

Start by walking short distances—two blocks is fine. Stop and rest if you need to. Don't risk injury by overdoing it; simply resolve to start small and work up to bigger and better things. Walking should be vigorous, so learn to swing your arms as you go. Breathe deeply and consistently. Do it regularly. Set aside some time each day for walking.

The Calories expended in walking range from 5 to about 8 per minute. Therefore, 40 minutes of walking uses from 200 to 320 Calories, depending on vigor, terrain, and your weight. As a rule of thumb, you should strive for 250 to 300 Calories per session, about four or five times each week. That comes down to 40 minutes each day.

Cycling

Bicycling at a moderate, safe speed consumes about 10 Calories per minute; 20 to 30 minutes spent cycling is excellent. It builds aerobic capacity with no pounding on any joints. It's got everything going for it and nothing against it.

Three-wheel bikes are now available for adults, which makes cycling possible at any age. In addition, cycling can become the transportation for shopping, errands, and socializing. It also has tremendous social value because anyone you meet on a bicycle already shares a common interest.

Swimming

Swimming is the best exercise of all. It places no stress on joints, it uses most of the muscle groups, and it's fun. To be effective, you should strive for about 30 minutes of nonstop swimming. There's no need to swim the fast crawl stroke shown on "Wide World of Sports"; just keep moving with a doggie paddle, breaststroke, backstroke, or sidestroke. If you can eventually knife through the water like a sea otter, excellent. You will have made my day. Simply be realistic: do it regularly for about 30 minutes and you will have achieved excellence.

Sports Activities

Tennis is great, but golf is one way to ruin a good walk. Golf is fine for recreation, but is not a good form of exercise. There are many recreational sports that have merits. Think through each one to see whether it provides vigorous activity for 20 to 40 minutes. If it does, then it's excellent; if not, do it for social purposes and choose serious exercise at other times.

Mechanical Bicycles and Other Devices

Through the marvels of modern engineering you can exercise regularly in the privacy of your home. All of these devices provide exercise with no jarring of joints and bones, with complete safety, and with convenience. Simply remember that you get what you pay for; it's better to spend more money for a machine that will last.

Exercise bicycles emphasize the legs. Get one on which you can adjust the tension so your output can reach your capability. The advantage is that you can read, listen to the radio, or watch television while doing it. This helps to alleviate boredom and can be an educational experience.

Rowing machines are very good because the better ones allow for leg, arm, and hip activity at the same time. They increase upper-body tone a little more than lower body, which is good because we tend to use our legs more in daily activity.

Rowing machines use from 10 to 15 Calories per minute, so 20 minutes, at low speed, should be the objective.

The Nordic Track is, in my opinion, the very best. It's what I use. It simulates cross-country skiing, which exercises, in a beneficial way, both the upper and lower body. The Nordic Track requires a little practice to get started, but even that will help your coordination. You can adjust both leg and arm-resistance for personal capacity and objective. It can be set to consume from 8 to 15 Calories per minute, depending on the speed you use.

Jogging

If you're a jogger, you should already be doing all the proper limbering and stretching exercises. Consider, though, that jogging places stress on all the weight-bearing joints, the back, and even the shoulders. It should be done in moderation by people with IBD.

Afterthoughts

This chapter is by no means comprehensive. There are as many forms of exercise as there are recreational activities. My objective is to get you started on limbering, stretching, and some regular activity. The benefits are so great that exercise usually gains its own momentum.

I urge everyone to purchase one of the many books on the subject, join a local group, or participate through radio, television, or by video rental.

Exercise and IBD

I've met professional athletes who have IBD. One of the cheerleaders in our local school has IBD. People with IBD jog regularly; in fact, I've jogged with two of them. Janet runs. Let her tell it: "I run about 35 miles per week. I've been doing it for the last 13 years!" Janet went on to explain that she's had surgery and has used prednisone, Flagyl, and bentyl. She's now off all medication and uses supplements, especially iron, which she takes because she had anemia. "At one point my iron level was one!" Janet's exercise program is excellent and she attributes much of her present health to it. Her correspondence with me indicated a very positive outlook. I believe exercise is a form of medicine. Don't say you can't exercise—you can! How you start is important. Start slowly and work up to whatever is good for you. Remember three things; in fact put them on your goal board:

- Thirty minutes each day for exercise! Find it; you've got it!
- Start slowly; you're only competing with yourself.
- Renew and revise your exercise goal every three months.

Success Loves Company

A recent study proved a point about success in exercise programs. It proved that success loves company. The most successful adults, by about 50 percent, were those who exercised as a husband-and-wife team. Most people who approach it with a spouse or close friend show similar success. The marriage vows say "for better or for worse"; they should add "with aerobics."

CHAPTER TWENTY-FOUR

Super Nutrition and Personal Experiences

I have a collection of questionnaires and letters that people have sent me telling about themselves. Most interesting was their response to my request for "additional comments." Some people were kind enough to send many pages of single-spaced typing; others made only a few comments. When I put them together, an interesting story unfolds.

Super Supplementation

Supplementation use ranged from none through some obvious misconceptions, to others who take lots of supplements.

Hanna, after a gradual buildup, takes the following supplements every day:

Children's chewable (about 25% adult RDA)	8
Alfalfa	16 or more
B Complex (450% RDA for all except	

folic acid and biotin)	7
Calcium (35% RDA)	4
Zinc (100% RDA)	6
Vitamin C (500 mg)	12
Vitamin E (400 I.U.)	6
EPA (omega-3, 270 mg)	3 (500 mg EPA daily)
Beta carotene (5,000 I.U.)	3
Protein supplement	48 grams daily

Mrs. Arthur O.: Although the amounts are unspecified, she takes a multivitamin-multimineral (50% RDA) in the morning and evening. In addition, she takes vitamin C, vitamin E, iron, alfalfa, Daily Fiber Blend, omega-3 oils, beta carotene, calcium, and B complex. She adds that the alfalfa stopped the bleeding and her doctor is impressed with how the scars on her intestine have healed.

Anette: "Metamucil helps if you take it before bedtime. My doctor recommended it and it works!" In addition, Anette uses the following:

Multivitamin-multimineral
Vitamin C (3,000 mg)
Iron
Beta carotene
Calcium (1,800 mg)
Potassium (75 mg)
Charcoal for gas

Hanna, Mrs. Arthur O., and Anette are typical of many people. However, most people used a much more moderate supplement program. Here's a few typical examples.

ALISON: Multivitamin, iron, and Metamucil daily.
GAIL: Multivitamin, Lactaid, and Metamucil.
MICHELLE: Multivitamin-multimineral about four times weekly.
JANET: "Woman's formula" and vitamin E; a B_{12} shot each month.
JOHN: Multivitamin prescribed by doctor.

TOM: Multivitamin once a day; Metamucil once a month.
RANDOLPH: Multivitamin daily and vitamin C monthly.

Many took a multivitamin regularly. A few, only four out of 100, didn't take any. As one woman put it so succinctly: "I don't believe in anything for this disease; it's like death!"

Heavy supplement users seemed to have more positive outlooks; they were enthusiastic. Most said that their doctors were generally satisfied with their progress. Some seemed especially pleased with their results after surgery.

I am concerned that about 25 percent of the people don't take a multivitamin with minerals. I encourage everyone to review chapters Eighteen through Twenty. Some people, on the advice of their physician, take a folic acid supplement. This is excellent; however, it would be more effective if it was taken along with a multivitamin-mineral supplement. It's essential to get all the nutrients at the RDA level every day. Just one or two vitamins and minerals aren't enough because no one, not even an expert, can be that precise about individual nutritional needs. Teamwork in nutrition is absolutely important.

My impression is that heavy-supplement users take medication at a lesser level than those who don't use supplements. People who use many supplements try to take more control over their own health. Many of them worked very hard, with their doctors, to reduce medication to a minimum. While this takes considerable effort, it's worthwhile. For example, if you can keep your dosage of prednisone to a minimum, you've done yourself a great service. I'm sure your doctor would agree.

Complaints about medication were about the same. No one likes to take prednisone; most people want to reduce it to a minimum. Some try and succeed!

Medication

Everyone hates the steroids. However, those with ulcerative colitis point out that it stops bleeding; those with Crohn's say that it stops diarrhea during a flare-up. Some people are very precise and can give the exact milligrams of prednisone needed to stop bleeding. They did it by working with their doctor and keeping a precise record of how they reacted to the medication.

Many people stay off medication as a result of successful surgery. Many other people, even after surgical removal of from a third to two-thirds of the small intestine, take from 8 to 16 separate medications daily. (I didn't know anyone could take that many different medications on a daily basis. It would be almost impossible to determine the side effects. It would be hard enough to keep track of when each one should be taken, let alone sort out your reactions.)

Side effects of drugs range from dizzy spells and wide mood swings to severe headaches. The word *headache* is mine and is probably inaccurate, because many people described it as Jean did: "My eyes get blurry and my head feels queer. It's hard to think." That's not the description of the average headache! Dry mouth is also common. Other people report that they experience no side effects even though they take from four to six different medications daily.

Prednisone receives the most complaints. Gail put it most clearly: "In October I started with 60 milligrams of prednisone, and every time the dosage was reduced I had problems. In January, I began to display psychological problems that were attributed to the high dosage. In February, they reduced the dosage to 30 milligrams daily. Now, one year later, I'm down to 5 milligrams every other day."

Azulfidine can cause kidney stones. Diane became quite angry about it. "I blame Azsulfidine for a large kidney stone; no one ever told me to drink lots of water with that drug." Reread Chapter Fifteen for help.

After reading all the comments and commentary, I strongly

urge people with IBD to discuss side effects openly with their physicians and pharmacists and to use reference materials. A diary will help the doctor sort out the side effects and develop the best program. It also helps to discuss side effects with peers at support group meetings. Person-to-person discussion can put them in a much clearer perspective.

One other problem that has emerged is the "generic" drugs. Both doctors' and patients' reports imply that they don't always produce the same results and they cause different side effects. The best solution is to keep a record of how you feel in the food diary, and discuss it with the doctor or pharmacist. Don't take chances!

Surgery

Many people are very positive about surgery.

Hanna's story is very touching; her Crohn's disease flared on her wedding day. She had to live at her parents' home for seven months after the wedding, seeing her husband only on weekends. After surgery, she says it in one clear statement: "Greatly improved by surgery; Allan and I were finally together." Hanna is the most positive of all and a heavy supplement user.

Fred had 2 feet of large intestine removed and more than 8 feet of small intestine. In his own words: "I can eat more foods now, but I must avoid foods that trigger a flare-up; I still have the disease. Attitude counts for a lot; a person cannot give up."

Jim has had his colon, rectum, large bowel, and all but 10 feet of small intestine removed. He says, "Surgery has reduced the foods I can eat by 50 to 75 percent." Jim is taking six different medications daily and goes on to conclude: "Now I have it in the lower third of my stomach. When the medication stops working, I'll need another operation." Jim will probably require TPN eventually.

Surgery produces many benefits. Some people can live a normal life and eat anything. For many others, surgery seems only to reduce the problems, so they're more manageable. It helps them live a more normal life. Surgery doesn't mean the end to medication. Indeed, many people, like Jim, continue taking five to six medications daily after surgery.

Alfalfa

A number of people who wrote to me about their IBD used supplemental alfalfa. Most people think of alfalfa as food for horses, but no horses corresponded with me. However, I did some research on alfalfa to learn more about its use as a food and a food supplement.

Alfalfa originated in what was called Persia and appears in writings concurrent with the Old Testament. That gives it a 7,000- to 10,000-year history. It is a pulse and is possibly one of the "pulses" referred to by Daniel in the Old Testament. Daniel and King Nebuchadnezzar conducted what could be called the first nutrition experiment proving the value of a vegetarian way of life. Pulse was specifically mentioned and was probably a dietary staple.

Alfalfa was largely used as human food in those days, since its leaves are nourishing and keep indefinitely when dried. It's a good source of protein, vitamins, minerals, and fiber. Over the years it acquired the name "medic," implying therapeutic properties. It slowly evolved into a silage crop because its unusually deep roots pull minerals to the surface; it promotes growth of nitrogen-fixing bacteria and consequently improves the quality of the soil. It's excellent feed for domestic animals with its rich protein and minerals. Human use relied largely on the dried leaves until about the early 1950s, when health food purveyors compressed it into tablets. From then until the present, it has been sold as a food supplement, but it is actually a food. After all, most tablets are nothing but compressed dried alfalfa leaves; sometimes with a little mint oil.

In my opinion, the benefits people get from alfalfa are

derived from its fiber content. Alfalfa contains soluble fiber and was used in some of Ershoff's studies (see Chapter Fourteen) to detoxify toxic materials in animals studies. The problem is quantity. If you were eating dried alfalfa leaves for fiber, you'd require about an ounce (e.g., 30 grams) to get a significant amount of fiber. Since alfalfa tablets contain about 300 milligrams of alfalfa, you'd need to take 20 to 40 tablets to get enough fiber to have a significant impact on your intestinal tract. But since most people don't get very much fiber, even fewer than 20 tablets would probably be noticed. In view of the comments about tablets, however, it would seem best for many people to chew the alfalfa tablets.

One problem mentioned by people with IBD is that tablets and capsules often pass through intact without dissolving. Others claim that any tablets irritate their intestine and cause trouble. Therefore, they chew their food supplements or use one of the liquid supplement foods. For that reason, I recommend that if you decide to experiment with alfalfa, the tablet should be chewed.

Mental Stress

Everyone who wrote identified "stress" as causative of flare-ups. Although I discussed stress in Chapter Twenty-two, I want to point out a few characteristics of the emotional stress they describe.

SUSAN: Learn to control yourself. "It didn't take long for me to see the pattern between the cramps, diarrhea, and stress. Once I saw the connection, I worked on my reactions to life. I did the following:

1. Stop trying to control.
2. Stop taking on other people's troubles.
3. Stop trying to do everything perfectly; accept doing as well as I can.

4. Stop sweating the small stuff; remember it's all small stuff."

Without knowing it, Susan is on her way through a program to controlling stress through the Alanon 12-step program. It seems to me that she and a few others could develop a similar program for IBD.

Tom pointed out something about IBD that is important: very few people understand the illness. Tom has been hospitalized several times, but so far has avoided surgery. He believes his success is in controlling stress together with family support.

My family gives me much support. I wouldn't have survived without my wife and support from family and friends. There are a lot of people that do not understand IBD and that makes it harder. You miss a lot of work, have to cancel get-togethers, etc. You start to look antisocial. People need to understand.

I was impressed by what Tom said. The solution could begin with more programs for families and friends of people with IBD, a short video about the disease that those with IBD could purchase and loan to friends, or support groups could maintain for loan.

RANDOLPH: "I feel fortunate that my case has remained fairly mild. The flare-ups I get are usually brought on by stressful situations. The fear that my illness may get worse is more debilitating than the illness itself."

ANETTE: Fear; inconvenience. "I'm afraid to go shopping or to a meeting with other women. I'm always afraid I'll ruin it for everyone because I'll get a flare-up."

ALISON: Medication (sulfa, prednisone, Flagyl, and others during flare-ups). "I have a round face, red nose, icky taste in my mouth, and night sweats. Every time we try to reduce the prednisone I get sick. I'm afraid I'll have to go like this for life." (Alison is under 30 years of age).

An awesome fear is the progression of IBD. It's similar to trying to satisfy a blackmailer who keeps asking for more. *Michelle*, a beautiful young lady who has already had a temporary colostomy, said it nicely: "The longer I have my disease, each flare-up becomes more difficult to treat. The symptoms do not subside as rapidly. Even after surgery, my IBD is still active. This current flare-up has lasted eight months." Michelle goes on to say she's been put on one more medication in hopes that it is the answer.

These four people represent many others living with IBD. Even though it seems bad already, there is the constant threat that it will get worse. It makes life inconvenient and if you're at all considerate of others, you can easily become reclusive about going places and socializing with others. Medication that helps people lead a more normal life has its side effects. But worse, the medication creates a fear all its own: the fear that you'll never be able to do without it. It's a double whammy because many people who have had surgery are taking as much medication as they did before the surgery. All this adds up to more stress.

I'll end with the comments of *Bob*, a man who has been treated by a physician using both nutrition (supplements) and medication (Azulfidine and other drugs). "Although several doctors told me that stress doesn't cause IBD, I believe that stress is a major cause from my own experience."

Some confusion has emerged. The basic cause of IBD remains unknown. Stress and emotional upset definitely have an influence on flare-ups, however, including the original flare-ups that led to the primary diagnosis. Stress that results from the disease and the side effects of medications cannot be discounted. Many people live a near normal life after surgery, but others don't. For them, surgery hasn't solved the problem. In some cases it has made life even more inconvenient.

An Alternative Treatment

Janet, twenty-seven, told me she has been on an experimental drug for six years. I'll use her words:

> I have been taking an experimental drug called Coherin for six years and stopped all other drugs except prednisone. I tried to stop taking Coherin this year. After I was off it for a couple of days I got very sick. For example, I wasn't able to eat, was tired, my stomach was bloated, and it hurt. Since I've been taking Coherin, I still get flare-ups, but the intensity is *much* less.

Janet has also taken prednisone daily for ten years. She started on Coherin six years ago and eliminated the other drugs. She points out that her flare-ups result from being overtired, stress, and eating large meals instead of many small meals. After receiving her correspondence, I decided to look into Coherin. I'll summarize what I've learned.

Coherin: An Experimental Drug

Coherin has been granted an investigational drug permit. This allows qualified physicians to give Coherin to IBD patients with their informed consent and understanding that they are taking an experimental drug. This means the investigators have met standards of safety and efficacy required by the U.S. Food and Drug Administration Bureau of Drugs. In this case side effects are insignificant.

Coherin is a polypeptide isolated from the posterior pituitary gland of cattle. A peptide is a "small protein," that is, a chain of special amino acids similar to a protein, not large enough to be so classified. The pituitary gland, located in the head, produces hormones and other substances that regulate many body activities. Coherin has definite physiological effects on animals and probably on people.

Coherin got its name from investigators, who claim it changes intestinal activity from a disorganized state to a organized pattern. In a sense, intestinal activity goes from incoherent to coherent; hence the name Coherin. Investigators of the drug claim that it brings on remission of inflammation. This is an unexpected finding because it means the abnormal, spastic activity of the intestine causes a certain amount of inflammation. This is contrary to the currently accepted hypothesis and, as a result, the drug is frowned upon by many research and practicing physicians.

The investigators claim that about 90 percent of the people who use Coherin get some benefit, whereas 10 percent get no benefit. Approximately 10 percent of the people who use it go into complete remission; 40 percent require Coherin daily and 40 percent intermittently.

Drs. Hiatt and Goodman, the investigators, concluded that Coherin has no discernible side effects. They also claim that it can be used to the exclusion of other medications with the exception of prednisone. They also point out that by taking Coherin, most patients can reduce prednisone levels significantly. Janet is a good example.

Is Coherin Effective?

If Coherin is effective it will require a significant clinical study in a major medical center. A drug company would have to produce the drug, underwrite the research, and publish results on a significant number of volunteer patients. Unfortunately, the fact that this hasn't been done doesn't mean it's not effective; it only means that funds aren't available, that other scientists are insufficiently interested to seek government funding, or they don't believe the results. Unfortunately, funding is often dictated by the number of people who have the illness and how protected the company will be that manufactures the drug. If Coherin can't be patented by the company that makes it, there's little financial incentive. If that's the case, research will have to rely on the Coherin Foundation, founded by Drs. Hiatt and Goodman with the objective of making the drug available and conducting research or government funding.

If you are interested in using Coherin, ask your doctor. Physicians must evaluate the results; if it's found to be ineffective or there is only a "placebo" effect, that also needs to be verified.

One Remedy for Flare-ups

Diane has a method of stopping the cramps that accompany her flare-ups. She found out about it from another friend who used it. I'll quote directly from her:

Soak a piece of flannel (to fit abdomen) in castor oil. Put it over abdomen. Cover with plastic (e.g. Saran Wrap). Place a heating pad over this; wrap and pin a large towel all around the abdomen. Turn heat pad on for 1–2 hours. Repeat several times a day and then taper off. You can reuse the oil-soaked flannel by just storing it (in a plastic bag) in the refrigerator. Sounds crazy, but it stops cramping. It's not a cure; I still had to have surgery a second time.

Weight: Good News

If IBD has a positive side it's that people who have it don't seem to be overweight. In fact, many people talk about sudden weight loss causing anxiety and worry. Any serious and sudden weight loss is cause for concern. If you know why it happened—for instance, as a result of a flare-up—you're in control. But if you don't, you should discuss it with your physician because it can be a symptom of a serious underlying problem.

Many people asked me how to determine a good weight. I use a rule that's easy to learn and works for most people. It goes as follows:

1. Measure your height in inches and subtract 60 (5 feet).
2. Multiply the remainder in inches by 5.
3. Women add the result to 100.
   Men add the result to 110.
4. You should be within about 10 percent of the number, depending on body type.

Take two examples: A woman 5 feet 5 inches and a man 5 feet 10 inches.

Woman 5″ × 5 = 25 + 100 = 125 with a 12-pound range
Man 10″ × 5 = 50 + 110 = 160 with a 16-pound range

Body type can be evaluated by evaluating neck size. If you have a long, slender neck, you should be close to the target; if you have a short neck, or if your head seems to grow right out of your shoulders (like the actor Danny DeVito), you will be closer to the upper limit.

My Own Thoughts on IBD

In my opinion, IBD will be found to be one of several variations of rheumatoid arthritis. Remember, there are about 100 variations of arthritis. They all have a hereditary predisposition and are probably related to a virus or bacterial infection that occurred long before the disease started or was diagnosed. The observation that a number of people must take as many as four to eight different medications daily, including prednisone, indicates that IBD isn't a single, simple illness. If results with Coherin are 30 to 50 percent positive, they indicate some significant variation in the disease.

Stress may not be a cause, but it reduces resistance and helps the process get started. Once established, emotional stress is clearly involved. It's a variation on an old question: Which comes first: IBD or the emotional stress? I'd like to see support groups focus on dealing with emotional stress.

Many people need a program that will help them like the one mentioned by Susan. It seems simple: just take one day at a time and learn to "let go." Unfortunately it isn't that easy for most people and they need help.

Education is essential. No, we don't require IBD education for everyone, but a short video and booklet for people who know someone with IBD, like schoolteachers, working associates, close friends, supervisors, and relatives, would relieve a lot of stress from misunderstanding. If those people close to a person with IBD understand the problems of the disease, it will help to relieve much of the emotional stress that accompanies this disease.

Suggested Reading

I have developed this list of suggested reading to satisfy diverse needs. It contains general information, as well as some important articles in medical journals that will lead the more technical-minded to entire libraries of information.

Complete Source of Information:

National Foundation for Ileitis and Colitis
444 Park Avenue South
New York, NY 10016-7374
1-800-343-3637

The foundation is an excellent reference for information on Inflammatory Bowel Disease. In addition to information, they sponsor education, support groups, and research.

Preface

The Crohn's Disease and Ulcerative Colitis Fact Book, Peter A. Banks, M.D., Daniel H. Present, M.D., and Penny Steiner, M.P.H., New York: Scribner, 1983.

The Arthritis Relief Diet, James Scala, Ph.D., New York: New American Library, 1988.

New Family Medical Guide, New York: Better Homes and Gardens, 1989.

The New Good Housekeeping Family Health and Medical Guide, New York: Morrow, 1989.

Your Gut Feelings, Henry Janowitz, M.D., New York: Oxford University Press, 1987.

"Economic Impact of Nutrition Counseling in Patients with Crohn's Disease in Canada," P. M. Baner et al., *J. of the Canadian Dietetic Assoc.* 49:236 (1988).

Treating IBD, Lawrence J. Brandt, Penny Steiner-Grossman, New York: Raven Press, 1989.

Chapter One

"Sulfite Sensitivity," R. A. Simon, *Annals of Allergy* 56 (4):281–291 (April 1986).

"Histamine in Foods: Its Possible Role In Non-Allergic Adverse Reactions To Ingestants," M. H. Malone and D. D. Metcalf, *NER Allergy Proceedings* 7 (3): 241–245 (June 1986).

"Dietary Aspects of Adverse Reactions To Foods in Adults," S. L. Parker, G. L. Sussman, and M. Krondl, *Canadian Medical Assoc. J.* 139 (8): 711–718 (Oct. 15, 1988).

"Possible Role of Food Sensitivity in Arthritis," R. S. Panush, *Annals of Allergy* 61 (6 Part II): 31–35 (Dec. 1988).

"Food Allergy and the Irritable Bowel Syndrome," *Am. J. Gastroenterology* 83 (9): 901–904 (Sept. 1988).

"The Roles of Inflammation and Iron Deficiency as Causes of Anemia," R. Yip and P. R. Dallman, *Am. J. of Clinical Nutrition* 48:1295 (1988).

"Nutrition Therapy for Rheumatic Diseases," R. S. Panush, *Annals of Internal Medicine* 106:619 (1987).

Physician's Desk Reference of Prescription Drugs, 43rd ed., Oradell, NJ: Medical Economics Inc., 1989.

The Essential Guide to Prescription Drugs, James W. Long, M.D., New York: Harper & Row, 1989.

Joe Graedon's The New People's Pharmacy #3, New York: Bantam, 1985.

Chapter Four

"The Acceptability of Milk and Milk Products in Populations with a High Prevalence of Lactose Intolerance," *The American J. of Clinical Nutrition* 48, October Supplement 1988.

The Milk Sugar Dilemma: Living With Lactose Intolerance, R. A. Martens, M.D., and S. Martens, M.S., R.D., Medi-Ed Press, 1987, P.O Box 957, East Lansing, MI 48826–0957.

Chapter Five

"Controlled Multi Centre Therapeutic Trial of An Unrefined Carbohydrate Fibre Rich Diet in Crohn's Disease," J. K. Ritchie et al., *British Medical Journal* 295:(517), Aug. 29, 1987.

"Fibre and Carrageenan in Inflammatory Bowel Disease," J. S. Whittaker and H. J. Freeman, *American J. Gastroenterology* 2 (Suppl. A): 38A–45A (Sept. 1988).

"Crohn's Disease and Ulcerative Colitis; A Review of Dietary Studies with Emphasis on Methodological Aspects," P. G. Persson et al., *Scandinavian J. Gastroenterology* 22 (4):385–389 (1987).

Chapter Six

Bowes and Churches Food Values of Portions Commonly Used, 15th Edition, Jean A. Pennington, Philadelphia: Lippincot, 1989.

Chapter Seven

"Vitamin Preparations as Dietary Supplements and Therapeutic Agents," Council on Scientific Affairs, *J. American Medical Assoc.* 257 (1929) April 10, 1987.

"Vitamin Supplement Use," G. Block et al., *American J. Epidemiology* 127(2):297–309 (Feb. 1988).

Chapter Eight

"The Cost of Home Total Parenteral Nutrition," R. J. Baptista et al., *Nutrition in Clinical Practice* 2 (1) 14 (1987).

"Small Intestinal Absorption and Tolerance of Enternal Nutrition in Acute Colitis," S. S. C. Rao et al., *British Medical Journal* 295 (698) Sept. 19, 1987.

"Enternal and Parenteral Nutrition," M. Irving, *British Medical J.* 291 (6506) 1404–1407, Nov. 16, 1985.

Chapter Nine

Diverticular Disease of the Colon, N. S. Painter, M.D., London: Heineman, 1975.

Chapter Ten

Jane Brody's Nutrition Book, Jane Brody, New York: Bantam, 1987.

Chapter Thirteen

"Clinical Aspects of Sucrose and Fructose Metabolism," J. Bantle, *Diabetes Care* 12:56 (1989).

Chapter Fourteen

"Effect of Dietary Fiber on Metabolizable Energy of Human Diets," C. W. Mills et al., *J. of Nutrition* 118:1075 (1988).

"Dietary Fiber Intake in the U.S. Population," E. Lanza et al., *Am. J. of Clinical Nutrition* 46(5):790–797 (Nov. 1987).

"Dietary Fiber Content of Selected Foods," J. W. Anderson and S. R. Bridges, *J. Clinical Nutrition* 47(3):440–447 (Mar. 1988).

"Health Aspects of Vegetarian Diets," *Am. J. Clinical Nutrition* 48(3 Suppl.):712–738 (Sept. 1988).

Medical Aspects of Dietary Fiber, edited by G. A. Spiller, and R. M. Kay, New York: Plenum, 1980.

Refined Carbohydrate Foods and Disease, D. P. Burkitt and H. C. Trowell (eds), London: Academic Press, 1975.

"Antitoxic Effects of Plant Fiber," B. H. Ershoff, *Am. J. Clin. Nutr.* 27: 1395 (1974).

Chapter Fifteen

"Prevention of Renal Stones by a High Fluid Intake," S. Ljunghall et al., *European J. Urology* 14(5):381–385 (Sept.–Oct. 1988).

Chapter Sixteen

"Vitamin K Deficiency in Chronic Gastrointestinal Disorders," *Nutrition Review* 44 (1):10–12 (Jan. 1986).

"Carotenoids in Human Blood and Tissues," R. S. Parker, *J. of Nutrition* 119:109 (1989).

Chapter Seventeen

"Loss of Vitamin C in Vegetables During the Food Service Cycle," B. L. Carlson et al., *European J. Urology* 14(5): 381–385 (Sept.–Oct. 1988).

"Recommended Dietary Allowances for Vitamins," V. Herbert, *J. of American Medical Assoc.* 260:1242 (1988).

Chapter Twenty

"Zinc in Growth and Development and Spectrum of Human Zinc Deficiency," A. S. Prasad, *J. of the American College of Nutrition* 7:385 (1988).

Chapter Twenty-one

"Oral Rehydration Therapy," A.K.C. Leung et al., *J. of The Royal Society of Health* 107:64 ff 1987.

The High Blood Pressure Relief Diet, J. Scala, Ph.D., New York: New American Library, 1989.

The K-Factor, Richard D. Moore, M.D., Ph.D., and George D. Webb, Ph.D., New York: Macmillan, 1986.

Chapter Twenty-two

"52 Minutes to Turn Your Life Around," David Viscott, M.D., Tape #307, Inner World Audio Publishers, 6115 Selma Ave., Los Angeles, CA 90028, (213) 467-5989.

The Joy of Stress, Peter G. Hanson, M.D., Kansas City/ New York: Andrews, McMeel and Parker, 1986.

Chapter Twenty-three

Aerobic Walking, Casey Meyers, New York: Vintage Books, 1987.

The Aerobics Program for Total Well Being, Kenneth H. Cooper, New York: Bantam, 1982.

APPENDIX

U.S. Recommended
Daily Allowances
(R.D.A.) 1989

FOOD AND NUTRITION BOARD, NATIONAL ACADEMY OF SCIENCES—NATIONAL RESEARCH COUNCIL
RECOMMENDED DIETARY ALLOWANCES,[a] Revised 1989

Designed for the maintenance of good nutrition of practically all healthy people in the United States

Category	Age (years) or Condition	Weight[b] (kg)	Weight[b] (lb)	Height[b] (cm)	Height[b] (in)	Protein (g)	Fat-Soluble Vitamins Vita-min A (µg RE)[c]	Vita-min D (µg)[d]	Vita-min E (mg α-TE)[e]	Vita-min K (µg)	Water-Soluble Vitamins Vita-min C (mg)	Thia-min (mg)	Ribo-flavin (mg)	Niacin (mg NE)[f]	Vita-min B6 (mg)	Fo-late (µg)	Vitamin B12 (µg)	Minerals Cal-cium (mg)	Phos-phorus (mg)	Mag-nesium (mg)	Iron (mg)	Zinc (mg)	Iodine (µg)	Sele-nium (µg)
Infants	0.0–0.5	6	13	60	24	13	375	7.5	3	5	30	0.3	0.4	5	0.3	25	0.3	400	300	40	6	5	40	10
	0.5–1.0	9	20	71	28	14	375	10	4	10	35	0.4	0.5	6	0.6	35	0.5	600	500	60	10	5	50	15
Children	1–3	13	29	90	35	16	400	10	6	15	40	0.7	0.8	9	1.0	50	0.7	800	800	80	10	10	70	20
	4–6	20	44	112	44	24	500	10	7	20	45	0.9	1.1	12	1.1	75	1.0	800	800	120	10	10	90	20
	7–10	28	62	132	52	28	700	10	7	30	45	1.0	1.2	13	1.4	100	1.4	800	800	170	10	10	120	30
Males	11–14	45	99	157	62	45	1,000	10	10	45	50	1.3	1.5	17	1.7	150	2.0	1,200	1,200	270	12	15	150	40
	15–18	66	145	176	69	59	1,000	10	10	65	60	1.5	1.8	20	2.0	200	2.0	1,200	1,200	400	12	15	150	50
	19–24	72	160	177	70	58	1,000	10	10	70	60	1.5	1.7	19	2.0	200	2.0	1,200	1,200	350	10	15	150	70
	25–50	79	174	176	70	63	1,000	5	10	80	60	1.5	1.7	19	2.0	200	2.0	800	800	350	10	15	150	70
	51+	77	170	173	68	63	1,000	5	10	80	60	1.2	1.4	15	2.0	200	2.0	800	800	350	10	15	150	70
Females	11–14	46	101	157	62	46	800	10	8	45	50	1.1	1.3	15	1.4	150	2.0	1,200	1,200	280	15	12	150	45
	15–18	55	120	163	64	44	800	10	8	55	60	1.1	1.3	15	1.5	180	2.0	1,200	1,200	300	15	12	150	50
	19–24	58	128	164	65	46	800	10	8	60	60	1.1	1.3	15	1.6	180	2.0	1,200	1,200	280	15	12	150	55
	25–50	63	138	163	64	50	800	5	8	65	60	1.1	1.3	15	1.6	180	2.0	800	800	280	15	12	150	55
	51+	65	143	160	63	50	800	5	8	65	60	1.0	1.2	13	1.6	180	2.0	800	800	280	10	12	150	55
Pregnant						60	800	10	10	65	70	1.5	1.6	17	2.2	400	2.2	1,200	1,200	320	30	15	175	65
Lactating	1st 6 months					65	1,300	10	12	65	95	1.6	1.8	20	2.1	280	2.6	1,200	1,200	355	15	19	200	75
	2nd 6 months					62	1,200	10	11	65	90	1.6	1.7	20	2.1	260	2.6	1,200	1,200	340	15	16	200	75

[a] The allowances, expressed as average daily intakes over time, are intended to provide for individual variations among most normal persons as they live in the United States under usual environmental stresses. Diets should be based on a variety of common foods in order to provide other nutrients for which human requirements have been less well defined. See text for detailed discussion of allowances and of nutrients not tabulated.

[b] Weights and heights of Reference Adults are actual medians for the U.S. population of the designated age, as reported by NHANES II. The median weights and heights of those under 19 years of age were taken from Hamill et al. (1979) (see pages 16–17). The use of these figures does not imply that the height-to-weight ratios are ideal.

[c] Retinol equivalents. 1 retinol equivalent = 1 µg retinol or 6 µg β-carotene. See text for calculation of vitamin A activity of diets as retinol equivalents.

[d] As cholecalciferol. 10 µg cholecalciferol = 400 IU of vitamin D.

[e] α-Tocopherol equivalents. 1 mg d-α tocopherol = 1 α-TE. See text for variation in allowances and calculation of vitamin E activity of the diet as α-tocopherol equivalents.

[f] 1 NE (niacin equivalent) is equal to 1 mg of niacin or 60 mg of dietary tryptophan. (Table used by permission.)

Index

Wheaties, 73
White blood cells, 305
Whitefish, 83
White vs. dark meat, 39, 84,
    157, 159
Whole-grain cereals, 41
Winged beans, 76
Women, 12, 13–14, 15, 23,
    93, 95, 99, 204, 229,
    255, 270, 282–83, 287,
    291, 293–94, 306

X

Xanax, 43
Xylitol, 59, 176, 178, 179
Xylose, 178

Y

Yambeans, 76
Yams, 36, 76, 223
Yautia, 76
Yeager, Chuck, 346
Yeast, 263, 264, 265, 266, 269
Yellow dye, 71
Yogurt, 24, 36, 58, 59, 61, 85,
    89, 99, 152, 159, 187, 280
Your Gut Feelings, 9

Z

Zinc, 5, 22, 31, 42, 43, 92, 93,
    105, 297, 299, 304–7, 310
Zucchini, 63, 88, 197, 208
Zyloprim, 43